TO BEAT...
...OR NOT TO BEAT?

Francisco Contreras, MD

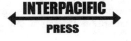

INTERPACIFIC
PRESS

To Beat...Or Not To Beat? By Francisco Contreras, MD
Published by Interpacific Press
1685 Precision Park Lane, Suite L
San Diego, CA 92173
Tel. (800) 950-6505
Tel. (619) 428-0930
Fax. (619) 428-0994

Editor: Daniel E. Kennedy
Copy Editor: Luisa Ruiz
Researcher: Jorge Barroso, MD, Ph.D.
Writing Staff: Michael Wood, Daniel E. Kennedy, Dr. Jorge Barroso, Luisa Ruiz, Dr. Jose Jimenez
Cover Design: Laura Monroy Amor and Daniel Kennedy
Graphic Art/Type Set: Laura Monroy Amor
Assistants: Gloria Rojo, Mary Bernal

International Standard Book Number: 1-57946-002-X

This book is not intended to provide medical advice or to take the place of medical advice and treatment from your personal physician. Readers are advised to consult their own doctors or other qualified health professionals regarding the treatment of their medical problems. Neither the publisher nor the author takes any responsibility for any possible consequences from any treatment, action or application of medicine, supplement, herb or preparation to any person reading or following information in this book. If readers are taking prescriptions medications, again, they should consult with their physicians and not take themselves off of medicines to start supplementation or nutrition program without the proper supervision of a physician.

Printed in the United States of America.

*To the philosophers, prophets and writers
who maintain that the heart is the seat
of the human soul.*

A LETTER

Dear John,

I realize that we are bound together until death do us part. Though I never had a say as far as who I wanted to be with, I have tried to make the best of it. I have been faithful to you, meeting all of your needs. Though our relationship has been one-sided, I have never complained. I have to speak up now, however, because I don't know how much more I can take.

At first I endured the things that you would do. You always insisted on eating foods that I don't like. When I wanted to get out and exercise, you would choose to sit around and expose me to smoke from your beloved cigarettes. That just kills me. I am speaking up now because the abuse you have dished out has passed the limit. Our relationship is no longer healthy and if things don't change soon, I will break down.

I agree that you are the brains in this relationship and that I am the working force of our enterprise, but please consider the fact that even a workaholic like me needs a good dose of TLC.

I am at your mercy but remember what the experts have told you. If you treat me right, I will be good to you. It is not too late to change your ways.

We can still get along together for many more happy years but you have to change. Otherwise, it is curtains for both of us. Don't take too long to make your decision. I am waiting and asking myself whether to beat....or not to beat? That is the question.

Sincerely,
    Your Heart

INTRODUCTION

This year I am celebrating my twentieth anniversary as a medical doctor. I, like most doctors, went into medicine because I wanted to help people. One of the most rewarding parts of my career has been writing books. Why? For one reason. I believe that the only true cure to disease is prevention. The beginning of prevention is knowledge. That's why books are so powerful. The field of medicine has made incredible advances in acute care but when it comes to chronic disease, we are still at square one.

Of all the books I have written, this may be the most important. Don't get me wrong. I think my books on cancer address a very serious issue but as far as heart disease goes, there is a lot more that people can do on their own to reverse it. It has been a personal mission of mine to go through medical literature, pull out the important applicable information and share it with the public. I have a wonderful research team that has helped me bring out some incredible facts. I am happy to say that this book is loaded with things that you can do to cut your risk of heart attacks down by 30 percent according to one study, 50 percent by another study and even 82 percent by the findings of another study. My hope as I write this book is that you will not merely read the book but that you will be motivated to put the information into action and add years to your life.

Let me give you an idea of how to navigate this book. If you like, you can read from beginning to end but you don't have to. You can go right to the parts that interest you most and then later pick up the rest. The chapters in this book are grouped by topic. The first seven chapters explain what heart disease is, what causes it and how it is affecting the general population. The next chapters focus on how to prevent and even reverse it. The chapters on healthy eating are the most important. Then there is a chapter that outlines the conventional heart care that is most frequently used. The final section goes into detail of a unique approach to heart care and prevention program. If you reference the table of contents your will be ready to roll.

I congratulate you on taking responsibility for your health by getting informed. It is my privilege to be a resource for you. Enjoy the book!

— Francisco Contreras, MD

TABLE OF CONTENTS

Dedication

A Letter

Introduction

1. Know Your Enemy 13

2. Friend Or Foe 19

3. Up In Smoke 25

4. Learning To Say No 28

5. Take A Load Off 38

6. Other Culprits 45

7. Back To Basics 48

8. A Healthy Appetite 52

9. Eat To The Beat Of A Different Drum 56

10. A Real Meal Deal 62

11. Get A Move On 74

12. Risky Business 79

13. Futuristic Therapies 83

14. State Of The Heart Health Care 86

15. Nature's Provision 94

16. Heart On Your Sleeve 104

References 110

Appendix I 133

Appendix II 136

Appendix III 145

Appendix IV 146

CHAPTER 1
Know Your Enemy

The first time I peered into a living body and was stunned by the marvel of a beating heart was in 1985. It was so beautiful it nearly brought me to tears. Unfortunately, the moment was ruined by my motive. The intensity of my interest was almost solely due to the astronomical rise in the incidence of heart disease in the mid-1900s. I knew that heart disease would be a formidable enemy to health in the years to come and I wanted to know my enemy.

Before 1900, heart disease was not nearly the threat it is today[1]. People exercised more regularly, usually because work demanded it, and they ate better, largely due to the absence of processed foods. In fact, the leading causes of death before 1900 were pneumonia and tuberculosis. Heart disease ran a distant fourth.

However, starting in 1901, heart disease began its meteoric rise and by 1910 was the leading cause of death in America. By 1959, heart disease claimed more lives than the next four causes of death combined.[2] By the late 1960s the World Health Organization called it the world's most serious epidemic.[3] It is still firmly entrenched in the top spot today.[4]

Without question, heart disease is the most serious threat to health in America. It is an equal opportunity killer of unparalleled proportions. It strikes men and women of every conceivable age, race, and status. It has not slowed in its meteoric rise to prominence. Every 33 seconds an American will die from heart disease.[5] Heart disease kills more people than the next seven causes of death combined. In 1997, close to a million Americans died from heart disease, twice as many as died from cancer, ten times as many as died in accidents, and fifty times as many as died from HIV.[6] More than one-third of the deaths that occur in the U.S. each year is from heart disease.[7] Americans wishing to live long and healthy lives should strive to understand this disease and how it may be prevented.

Caught in a Tight Spot
If you wrap a string tightly around a finger, that finger will quickly begin to turn purple. Soon, you will experience a very sharp pain. This same thing happens to your heart during a heart attack. Heart attacks occur because the most prevalent heart disease involves the vessels that feed the heart itself, the coronary arteries.

Nearly all coronary artery disease results from atherosclerosis. This term derives from two Greek words; *athero*, meaning "paste," and *sclerosis*, meaning "hardness."[8] You see, arteries are supposed to be flexible and smooth, but often deposits of fat and calcium, called plaque, build up on the inner walls.[9] When these plaques cause artery walls to harden and lose elasticity, a condition occurs called arteriosclerosis. Arteriosclerosis is atherosclerosis of the arteries. If unchecked, the plaque buildup can eventually block a coronary artery and cause a heart attack.[10]

Early studies in the 20th century revealed that atherosclerosis, the hardening of arteries, was the primary cause of heart disease. However, what shocked the medical world was how quickly arterial plaque formed. Studies of soldiers killed in the Korean War revealed that more than three-quarters had gross evidence

14

of heart disease. A similar study during the Vietnam War produced the same results. The average age of these soldiers was twenty-two.[11]

Arteriosclerosis does not only occur in the heart. When other major arteries develop blockages, other parts of the body are negatively impacted. Stroke, high blood pressure, abdominal pain, weight loss, muscle discomfort, ulcers, and even gangrene can occur because of arteriosclerosis.[12]

Tell Me Where It Hurts
Because of the epidemic proportions of this disease, people should have a working understanding of its symptoms. The most common symptom is a very specific type of chest pain, called *angina pectoris*. Angina pectoris is a feeling of pressure or heaviness in the center of the chest, the neck, the shoulder, the arm or lower jaw. This pain tends to gravitate toward the left side of the body. Angina pectoris also tends to occur after the heart has been "stressed."[13]

There are other types of pain that suggest infirmity, but not of the heart. If your chest discomfort lasts more than twenty minutes, you are either having a heart attack or you are not having heart problems at all. Sharp "stabbing" pain is usually not heart related pain, nor is pain that remains confined to a small area. [14]

Heart problems are difficult to diagnose because the symptoms are similar to less serious afflictions. Signs of a blocked coronary artery can be indigestion, nausea, bloating, belching, vomiting, shortness of breath, sweating, clammy skin, paleness, dizziness, fainting, and fatigue. While few people assume they have heart disease when they have indigestion or nausea, looking for an accumulation of symptoms is a wise habit to practice.

Under Attack
The heart attack is the last gasp of a diseased heart. Doctors call it acute myocardial infarction.[15] A heart attack occurs when blood

supply to the heart is restricted because of a blocked coronary artery. Less blood means less oxygen and when cells become starved for oxygen they begin to die.

The severity of a heart attack depends on where the heart is damaged. If an area critical to the heart's ability to function is damaged the attack can end in death. Blockages of some coronary arteries are more life-threatening than others.[16] However, a victim can survive when the affected area is less critical. [17]

At least 250,000 people die of heart attacks each year and those who survive have weakened hearts. A heart weakened by myocardial infarction will struggle to move blood through the body. Often, a damaged heart can not handle the workload. If this is the case, the heart eventually gives way to *congestive heart failure*. It is clear that when a heart suffers from prolonged disease it is often damaged beyond the point of repair.

Oh, The Things We Do To Ourselves
The cause of heart disease is still a controversial topic of discussion in the medical community. This is because there are a wide number of variables to consider. However, the primary factors are readily evident. I believe the choices we make and the habits we develop are the most important determining factors for heart disease. Basically, if we put the right things into our bodies and we exercise, we will greatly reduce the risk of heart disease. Whereas, if we put the wrong things into our bodies and we lack exercise, we will greatly increase the risk of heart disease.

According to the modern medical community, if we have high blood pressure, high cholesterol, or diabetes we are high-risk candidates for heart disease. Likewise, if we are obese we will hear the same. If we smoke cigarettes or drink alcohol to excess a doctor will look us in the eye and tell us that we are high-risk candidates. All of these factors can be attributed to what we put into our bodies. In addition, high blood pressure and obesity are also clearly linked to inactivity, or a lack of regular exercise.

While there remains some debate over other factors in the heart disease equation, this much seems clear. What we *choose* to put into our bodies and the exercise habits we *develop* will play a major role in determining the level of risk we live with year after year.

Pay Now or Pay Later

Some of the best advice my father ever gave me growing up was to learn to maintain the automobiles I owned. He recommended changing the oil and refilling the fluids every 3,000 miles, replacing the plugs every 5,000 miles, and checking the belts and rubber every 10,000 miles. I can tell you that those little maintenance pit stops dented my wallet sometimes, but my father's philosophy was simple. Either you pay now or you *pay* later. If you've ever had a car break down and had to take it to the shop, you know exactly what my father meant when he said *pay* later. Mechanics can work miracles, but they certainly don't perform them for free.

Pay now or *pay* later. This simple truth seems so obvious. Yet, when we are told the importance of preventive heart maintenance, often we adopt a let's-wait-and-see approach. Perhaps we choose to wait because we believe medical technology has taken the sting out of heart disease, or that nothing is irreversible anymore. This is not true.

It is true that tremendous technological advances have been made in the medical industry's fight against heart disease. Coronary arteriography, cardiac catheterization, echocardiography, angioplasty, atherectomy, coronary artery bypass graft surgery, heart transplant surgery, and artificial heart surgery are some of the major technological advances made in recent years. However, this technology may have lulled us into a false sense of security.

Think back to the automobile. Suppose we as car owners adopt a let's-wait-and-see approach to auto maintenance. This means that we do relatively nothing to the car until it breaks down. Then we take the car to the shop, sometimes we have it towed because it is no longer operable, and often we discover that there are parts that are beyond repair and that need to be replaced. We leave the shop and call the bank to take out a second on our home loan because we have glanced at the mechanic's estimate and the cost is larger than the gross national product of Zimbabwe.

You laugh, but we are proceeding in just this fashion where our hearts are concerned. Most of us do nothing to maintain it until it breaks down. Then we go to the shop, sometimes we are towed there because the heart is no longer operable, and often we discover that there are parts that are beyond repair and that need to be bypassed or replaced. If we think a mechanic's bill is steep, we are fooling ourselves. A heart surgeon's bill far surpasses it. And while people survive trips to the auto shop, there are plenty of people with heart disease who will not make it off the operating table.

We can not hide our heads in the sand any longer. We must learn to understand heart disease and begin to do the things that will maintain the health of our hearts. Remember the words of my father, pay now or *pay* later.

CHAPTER 2
Friend Or Foe?

In the Heart of Cajun Country

I can remember travelling to the city of New Orleans to give a lecture once. In the fading light of the late afternoon my wife and I stepped out into the French Quarter to enjoy a meal. There are many artists living in New Orleans and most of them are chefs. We sat down in a cozy little restaurant specializing in continental cuisine. As the waiter set my plate down, I looked at the bacon-wrapped filet mignon sitting on a bed of stilton cheese with aged balsamic vinegar drizzled over the crusted top. I reminded myself that it is not the occasional meal but the routine diet that makes or breaks a healthy lifestyle. Then, I ate to my heart's content.

I must admit. I also thought how hard it must be for those living in the area to abstain from cholesterol dense foods when surrounded by them. I was not shocked to discover later that New Orleans is the heart disease capital of the country. Studies show that heart disease rates in "food-rich" cities like New Orleans, Chicago, and New York, are significantly higher than the rest of the country.[1]

How ironic. That city sits at the mouth of the Mississippi River, the country's most significant "artery." As this river flows it picks up dirt particles, which it then deposits as sediment in the arterial web of the delta. Sediment impedes the unrestricted flow of water. In like fashion our blood stream picks up the impurities we ingest which it deposits as plaque along the walls of our arteries. Plaque impedes the unrestricted flow of blood to vital areas of the body. This process, called atherosclerosis, is traditionally linked directly to cholesterol. Let's find out more about this enemy to health.

A Bad Rap

Cholesterols are lipids, which are found in the blood. The mainstream medical community has established a firm link between many cholesterols and heart disease. Most people picture cholesterol as a yellow, oily sludge smeared along the inside of artery walls. In reality, such an image is more like fat than cholesterol. Cholesterols are pearl-colored, waxy, and solid. They feel like soap between the fingers.[2]

Most people also imagine that cholesterols come from fast food. Nothing could be further from the truth. Cholesterols are produced naturally by the body. They play a vital role in the natural maintenance of the body, just as enzymes, hormones, and blood cells do. In fact, without cholesterols we would die.

For one, cholesterols are the building blocks for the hormones estrogen and testosterone. They also help to form adrenal hormones, which help regulate blood pressure. Cholesterols aid in the digestion of fats and vitamins A, D, E and K. Cholesterols assist in the normal growth and repair of cells, particularly of brain cells. Cholesterols actually help transport blood fats through the circulatory system. In fact, cholesterol levels that are too low can mean the body is dying.[3]

An Endless Supply

More than 80 percent of a body's cholesterols are produced by the body. The liver is the primary factory and distribution center but individual cells are capable of producing their own cholesterols.

20

Almost 95 percent of a body's cholesterols are found in cells protecting cell membranes by regulating the elimination of waste and the absorption of nutrients. Surprisingly, only a small percentage of a body's cholesterols are found in the blood stream.[4]

Understand that a body needs large amounts of cholesterol to function properly. Because of this the body works extremely hard to maintain consistent cholesterol levels. This is why it is so hard to significantly lower cholesterol levels through diet.[5]

Two Sides of the Same Coin

Most modern medical doctors would have you believe that there are "good" cholesterols and "bad" cholesterols. They will explain in detail that high-density cholesterols (HDL) help protect your blood vessels against cardiovascular disease, by reversing cholesterol transport, which helps remove bad cholesterol from blood cells and arterial walls. They will say that HDL cholesterols are a major protective agent in the fight against atherosclerosis.

These same doctors will often assert that low-density cholesterols (LDL) cause inflammation of arterial walls. They will also claim that LDL cholesterols contribute to the buildup of fatty plaques and the thickening of the blood. They will state that LDL cholesterols are the prime suspect in the formation of dangerous blood clots. In short, the medical community generally views cholesterols as follows: the lower the density of the lipid, the more harmful the cholesterol is to our health.

There Are Two Sides to Every Story

Forgive me for flying in the face of conventional wisdom, but I find this black-and-white view of cholesterols terribly inadequate. It is difficult for me to believe that the body would produce harmful substances within the design of normal everyday function.

The human body is a wonderfully economical mechanism. There are no wasted steps or unnecessary processes. LDL cholesterols are a necessary element in the normal function of the

21

body. What makes these substances harmful is the same thing that makes most substances within the body harmful, that is, excess or deficiency. You see, there really is too much and too little of a good thing.

A healthy balance depends on the ratio between the two cholesterols rather than the overall quantity of each individually. Here is the quick and easy way to determine if a body has a healthy cholesterol balance. A minimum of 25% of the body's total cholesterol count should consist of HDL cholesterols. In addition, the body's LDL cholesterol count should never exceed three times that of its HDL cholesterol count.

Independently of how high or low your "cholesterol" is, if your ratios are within these numbers, your risk of suffering from heart disease is low. Conversely, no matter how low your total cholesterol is, if the ratios of LDL and HDL are higher than these two numbers, your risk of heart disease is much higher. Remember, ratio is more important than overall level. To calculate your cholesterol levels you can refer to appendix III or visit www.nutritionfacts.us

Playing by the Numbers
Doctors love numbers. There is a dependable comfort in numbers. Yet, numbers can be deceiving. Plenty of evidence suggests that no particular numerical level of cholesterol is "right" for people in general. Many doctors now argue that cholesterol levels are tailored to the individual. This was proven in 1998 by a team of scientists who discovered that "only a fraction of the cholesterol we consume is actually absorbed by the body" and that "different people absorb different amounts."[6]

Furthermore, it is widely known that laboratory equipment can make it difficult to measure cholesterol levels to any degree of certainty. After all, cholesterol tests are done on the blood, but only seven percent of the body's cholesterol is found in the blood. The rest is dispersed throughout the body.

To demonstrate the inaccuracy of modern lab equipment, a Wall Street Journal reporter sent blood samples to five different labs in New York and got back separate results placing him in high cholesterol, borderline-high cholesterol, and low cholesterol categories. Again, it is better to think about ratio first and worry about total cholesterol intake less.[7]

Guilty by Association

It has been suggested that dietary cholesterols, or those we consume in foods, may act synergistically with saturated fatty acids. While there is evidence demonstrating that saturated fatty acids dramatically increase LDL cholesterol levels in the body, there is little evidence connecting dietary cholesterols to the increase. Yet, it is generally recommended that both cholesterols and saturated fats should be restricted in the healthy diet. But should they?

Shepherds in Somalia eat almost nothing but milk from their camels, containing about a pound of fat per day. Yet, their cholesterol is much lower than in most western countries.[8] In many other cultures that consume primitive diets, no signs of arteriosclerosis or heart disease is found, even in the very old. The connection between diet and cholesterol level is debunked in these places and there are too many of them for scientist to pass it off as an anomaly.

U.S. studies confirm this. A recent study claimed that variations in blood cholesterol levels were in no way connected to diet and found that those with low blood cholesterol ate just as much saturated fat as those with high cholesterol. In fact, no evidence exists that too much cholesterol in the diet promotes heart attacks or hardening of the arteries.[9] Yet, Americans remain obsessed with the idea of lower cholesterol levels in an effort to prevent heart disease. We must focus our energies in other directions.

An Empty Promise

As the national frenzy over cholesterol levels continues, the public looks for the comfort of a quick fix. Enter the pharmaceutical

23

industry. Never one to pass up a golden opportunity, this industry has produced a staggering number of drugs designed to lower cholesterol levels. What is most insidious about this is the unspoken hope of consumers that these drugs are good preventative practice. However, we know that there is little connection between cholesterol level and heart disease.

Clinical trials showed that some of these drugs were very effective in bringing down cholesterol levels, but the "control" group had the better survival rate. Unbelievably, the group receiving a placebo had an almost thirty percent better survival rate! In another notorious study, called the Helsinki Heart Study, a cholesterol-lowering drug was administered to more than four thousand patients. The drug lowered cholesterol and the incidence of heart attack, but the control group still realized a better overall survival rate.[10]

While these drugs may save the lives of individuals whose cholesterol ratios are grossly out of balance, many times they are prescribed to people who do not need them. Do not forget that these drugs produce side effects. It is unconscionable to make such drugs widely available, to advertise them heavily in magazines and on television, and to give people the false impression that these drugs are an effective preventative measure.

Arteriosclerosis, the arterial sludge that acts like the dirty sediment of the Mississippi Delta, begins in childhood. This buildup of plaque in the arteries is caused by many factors, but we have ignored the key factors for far too long. Diet and exercise are the most powerful keys in the prevention of arteriosclerosis.

In the next few chapters we will examine some of the factors that have the most significant power to increase your risk of heart disease.

CHAPTER 3
Up In Smoke

You must know that smoking is bad for you. There is so much information and public service announcements about the hazards of smoking that I almost feel like those who blow smoke in the face of these warnings deserve to reap what they are sowing. Since smoking is obviously dangerous, I considered not writing about it. But I have to or this book wouldn't qualify as a heart book because tobacco smoking is the number one cause of heart disease. So, let's get to the subject.

Cigarettes consist of at least 43 different cancer-causing substances, and thousands of others that are capable of mutating our genes and poisoning our very bodies. A lot of people are aware of facts like this but they just won't change. I remember one patient that arrived at the Oasis of Hope Hospital. She was having such a fit in the reception that they had to call the Executive Vice President. She had arrived for lung cancer treatment but she grunted to the VP, "I won't talk to you until somebody gets me a cigarette."

The damage to our lungs caused by smoking is well-known, but less known is the damage it does to our hearts and circulatory system.

Let's take a look at some of the facts:

- 30 percent of heart disease deaths in the U.S. can be attributed to cigarette smoking. This according to the American Heart Association.[1]
- In 1990, 418,690 U.S. deaths were attributed to smoking of which 179,820 resulted from cardiovascular diseases, this according to the Centers for Disease Control.[2]
- Smoking affects the cardiovascular system lowering its ability to function under duress and it increases the risks associated with high blood pressure, high cholesterol, physical inactivity, obesity and diabetes.[3]
- Nicotine hardens arteries, causes blood clots, damages the cell lining of blood vessesl, increases blood pressure and heart rate, lowers the blood's capacity to deliver oxygen and causes blood to stick to artery walls.[4]
- Smoking a single cigarette may increase the formation of blood clots.[5]

I would like to see television producers fit all of that information into a public service announcement! So, if you smoke, will you be more likely to get heart disease? Yes. A pack a day doubles your risk of a heart attack. If you smoke, you have five times less probability of surviving a heart attack than a non-smoker does. There are only three things for sure in life.

1. Everyone has to pay taxes.
2. Everybody will die one day.
3. If you keep smoking after you have a heart attack, you will suffer a more serious heart attack in the future.[6]

Let's look at this from a different perspective. Each carton of cigarettes you smoke takes one and a half days off of your life. Let's get more dramatic. Every cigarette you smoke will shorten your life by 11 minutes.[7] Think about it, if you quit smoking, you will add years to your life to do things like spend more time with your kids.

26

Conclusion

I want to wrap this chapter up with a few more facts. Second-hand smoke is more dangerous than first-hand smoke. If you smoke, please don't do it around your children or your spouse. I have had patients die who never smoked but their husbands did. The husbands are so repentive for their actions. Imagine how parents who smoke feel when their children get cancer.

Also, cigars are just as damaging as cigarettes, even if you don't inhale. The truth is that you may not inhale initially but as the room you are in fills up with smoke, you start breathing second hand smoke. One study reported "Regular cigar smoking increases the risk of cardiopulmonary heart disease, chronic obstructive pulmonary disease, and cancers of the upper aerodigestive tract and lung. Individuals who smoke more than four cigars a day are exposed to an increased amount of smoke, the equivalent of ten cigarettes a day." [8]

Not only that, but cigars are unfiltered, meaning that the smoke from cigars has more nicotine, lead nitrogen oxides, ammonia, carbon monoxide and other devastating compounds than cigarettes. [9]

Another thing that really gets to me is how women's mortality from lung cancer and heart disease have increased since the feminist movement began. Women claimed rights not only in the area of work but also in the area of bad habits including smoking and drinking.

But take heart, all of this damage can be reversed. "As soon as you stop smoking," says one medical authority, "your body begins to heal itself from the devastating effects of tobacco." [10]

Twenty minutes after you stop smoking, your blood pressure goes back down. Within a day your chance of a heart attack decreases, and by two months your circulation improves. After a year, your risk of heart attack is half what it would have been had you continued smoking, and after two years it is almost the same as the risk of a non-smoker. [11]

27

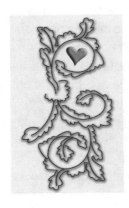

CHAPTER 4
Learning To Say "No"

Every child goes through that period where they test the waters of defiance. It is during this stage in life that their answer to everything will be "no." Ask them to pick up their room and you will get a "no" and an argument. I've noticed that some people never grow out of that stage. In fact, some people cultivate the behavior into an art form. We call those people curmudgeons. They argue for sport.

I have a friend like that—my best friend, in fact. This friend loves to point out that many people enjoy long and healthy lives while eating junk foods and fancy French cuisine. George Bernard Shaw said that, "There is no more sincere love than the love of food," and my friend is living proof of that. He is bent on proving his own theory that junk food is okay, and disproving my idea that diet greatly impacts health.

We do agree on some points, though barely. He agrees that exercise is important so he plays golf. I hold with Bob Hope who said, "If you watch a sport, it's fun. If you play it, then it's recreation. If you work at it, then it's golf." Exercise is important but I refuse to call golf exercise, especially since my friend drives a cart. In fact, the best exercise I get while golfing, is when I am wrapping my seven-iron around a tree trunk in frustration.

However, I try to keep my body in good shape. My friend, on the other hand, does not worry too much about keeping in shape. In fact, the only thing he keeps in perfect "shape" is his rounded belly. Still, he likes to point out that the only way we will settle the junk food debate is by seeing who dies first. It sounds morbid, but we actually argue over who is going to be speaking at the other one's funeral.

I have to admit that I don't know for sure that I will live longer than my friend, but I would not exchange my lifestyle in order to imitate his. I'm going to keep eating right because I know for a fact that life can be lengthened and enhanced if a person improves his or her diet. However, I do wish to imitate one aspect of my friend's character, and that is his ability to say "no."

The Art of Saying "No"

A big part of improving our diet is avoiding foods that harm our hearts. These days, that means rejecting much of what is considered normal by the society at large. Every day we are tempted by images of popcorn slathered in butter, fast food hamburgers sizzling over flames, french fries sprinkled with salt, etc. Yet, the simple truth is these foods are unhealthy because they contain so much fat and so little nutritional value.

These foods are unhealthy because they are processed and preserved to such an extent that they are hardly foods at all. Instead they are manufactured products that happen to be somewhat digestible. We must learn to say "no" to these foods if we want to protect our hearts from disease. The following are the eight key foods we must strive to avoid: foods containing refined sugar, foods containing refined flour, foods containing processed oils, foods containing too much salt, foods containing pesticides, foods that are fertilized, foods that are seasonally manipulated, and foods that are hormone-injected.

Be Sugar Free

If you had to guess which three foods are the staple of the American diet, what would you say they are? The answer is refined sugar, refined flour, and processed oils. These three ingredients form the basis of most of what the average American eats. Every cracker, cereal, pastry, fruit bar and most other snacks are made up of refined sugar, refined flour and processed oil. Do an experiment. Go into your pantry and look at the ingredients on the bags or boxes of food. You might be surprised how often these "three amigos" turn up.

Of the three, refined sugar is perhaps the most consumed food on the planet. Everything from fruit juice to candy bars to canned corn is sweetened with it. Think for a moment of what you have eaten today already. In all likelihood you have met your FDA recommended sugar intake.

Refined sugar is relatively new to the world scene. It was invented in 1751. Before then nobody ate refined sugar. Today the average American eats about 150 pounds per year. That works out to about half a pound a day![1] Imagine yourself sitting in front of a bowl spooning eight ounces of white sugar into your mouth. Get the picture?

Refined sugar is created when raw sugar is stripped of any substances that cause it to decompose. The sweet part of the sugar remains, but everything of nutritional value is gone. In fact, nutritionists call it an "anti-nutrient" because our bodies must waste nutrients in order to turn it into something useable.

What does this have to do with the heart? There is a direct relationship between the explosion of heart disease in this century and the skyrocketing consumption of refined foods. A diet that consists mainly of sugar can bring on many illnesses, and is believed to increase the risk of heart attacks.[2]

It has been shown that people who eat less sugar live longer. The Seventh Day Adventists, for example, eat a vegetarian diet and avoid refined foods. It is no coincidence that they live an average of twelve years longer than the rest of the population. Should we rule out all sweets? No. Nature provides a wonderful sweetener called honey, a naturally occurring, unrefined sweet-

30

ener that tastes every bit as good as sugar and won't harm our hearts.

I suggest replacing refined sugar with honey as often as you can. You can bake with honey, pour it into coffee or tea and spread it on bread. It has a rich, complex, sweet taste that makes refined sugar seem almost childish. You will enjoy it immensely, I assure you.

Flour Power

We will see later in the book how healthy grain and fiber are for the heart. But often we don't derive any benefits from wheat because most of it is refined. When grain is refined and turned into white flour it loses nearly all of its nutrients, and the number of calories goes up by seven percent! White flour is almost a non-food, virtually stripped of all nutritional value.

Even "enriched" breads are not truly healthy. They contain a few added vitamins and minerals, but not nearly enough to make up for what was lost in refining. Worse, refined flour and white breads are treated with chemicals and bleach that get inside our arteries and cause damage. You would do well to eliminate refined flours from your diet, as much as you can. If you want to experience flour power, make sure you choose the whole grain alternatives that are readily available in the supermarket.

Processed Oils

You have probably seen the words "partially hydrogenated vegetable oil" on a product in your cupboard or refrigerator. Partial hydrogenation is a process of heating vegetable oils to change their chemical constitution, producing a fat that is solid at room temperature. Margarine and shortenings are examples of these products. Many foods, particularly snack foods, contain partially hydrogenated fats.

Foods made with partially hydrogenated fats last longer than foods made with animal fats, and are less expensive. Yet these

31

chemical substances can't be metabolized by our body. Even worse, they block our body's use of essential oils.

Processed oils have been shown to increase the risk of heart disease. A study in a major medical journal said that, "Given the proper incentives, the food industry could replace a large proportion of the partially hydrogenated fats used in foods and food preparation with unhydrogenated oils. Such a change would substantially reduce the risk of coronary heart disease at a moderate cost."[3]

You should avoid processed oils and foods with the words "partially hydrogenated oil" on their label. Substitute olive oil and butter for margarine and Crisco. Leave the chemicals for the cleaning supply cabinet, not the pantry.

Salt of the Earth
I will never forget an encounter with an elderly Scandinavian couple at a dinner function in Los Angeles. We were served chicken for the main course and I could not help but notice what happened next. These lovely people each asked the waiter for a salt shaker. They then proceeded to put three to four shakes of salt on each bite they took. Each bite! I have never been so transfixed at the dinner table before.

The world is fascinated by salt. The history of salt is long, convering thousands of years. Early civilization was concerned with finding and conserving salt. It was so precious that social bonds were formed over it.[4]

Because salt is abundant in our diet and cannot always be tasted, it is difficult for us to know when we are overindulging ourselves. What should concern us is that most of our salt intake comes from processed food, where salt is used as a preservative and often is not tasted.[5] . Only 20 percent to 30 percent of total dietary sodium consumption is consumer-controlled through the addition of salt to food after its preparation. The rest is derived from naturally occurring sources or commercial processes.

It is widely known that hypertension plays an important role in the development of heart disease. What is still a source of debate is who, exactly, should restrict their intake of dietary salt and whether a low-salt diet is an effective treatment for hypertension.[6] My recommendation is that we all adjust our salt intake to moderate levels while the medical community makes up its mind.

To avoid excessive intake of salt, people should choose foods low in salt, like fresh fruits and vegetables, and avoid foods high in salt, particularly pre-prepared foods. People should also be aware of the salt content of food choices in restaurants.[7] Hypertensive patients, particularly those over the age of 44 years, should restrict their salt consumption to 3 to 6 grams of salt per day.[8] We are better safe than sorry, and the adjustment is not so extreme.

The War on Bugs

The food industry hates bugs and combats them with pesticides so that American consumers can have grocery stores lined with fruit that is cosmetically appealing, and that lasts weeks rather than days. In truth, "buggy" fruit is not really a threat to our health. Washing or cooking it takes care of that problem.

But pesticides are a huge public health threat. Mounting evidence says that exposure to them can cause cancer and other degenerative diseases. I am certain that someday tests will show a connection between heart disease and pesticides because of the damage these chemicals inflict on the lining of our arteries.

When food is treated with chemicals, those chemicals get inside our bodies and inflame the lining of our arteries, causing them to harden. It takes years, decades, lifetimes to rid the body of these chemicals. Instead of buying the strange-looking, too-perfect fruit and vegetables at the supermarket, seek out a store that sells pesticide-free produce. Look for the organic label. That way you can avoid putting those poisons into your blood stream.

Spoiled Soil

Fertilizers, too, damage the foods we eat. To grow the vegetables and fruits bigger and faster, growers dump indiscriminate amounts of fertilizers into the soil, and as soon as the harvest is done, the soil is prepared for the next crop. The nutritional value of the fruits and vegetables grown in fertilized soil is dramatically diminished.

The most frequently used fertilizers destroy iron, vitamin C, folic acid, minerals, lysine and many other amino acids, among other nutrients. If land were allowed to rest, it would retain its ability to give nutrition. Instead, growers use fields year-round, in and out of the natural season, and would never consider giving their fields an entire year off.

Again, eating organically-grown, fertilizer-free produce will help you to get the heart-healthy nutrients you need, and avoid the questionable chemicals that come with the fertilizer.

Ripe For The Picking?

To increase shelf life, farmers harvest fruits and vegetables long before they are mature, even though produce absorbs most of its vitamins and minerals when it is almost ripe. There is a time to plant and a time to pluck the fruit. This means that there is also a time not to pluck the fruit. But modern agriculture demands that the season always be "now."

Green bananas will never fill up with vitamins and minerals sitting on your kitchen counter! Potatoes lose most of their vitamin C in a week, and spinach greens, asparagus, broccoli and peas lose half of their vitamins before they get to market. Packaging and transportation compromises nutritional value even more. If picked and left outside more than two or three hours, nutritional value is further reduced. Frozen vegetables lose one-fourth of vitamins A, B1, B2, C and niacin. Broccoli, cauliflower, peas and spinach lose up to half of their vitamins. Canned foods lose more than half of all nutrients—but provide a substantial amount of lead!

Eating fresh, organically-grown produce is the best way to get nutrients. Seek out a farmer's market and inquire about their growing methods. Ask if they let their fields rest; if they use pesticides or fertilizers. With the growing popularity of organic foods, such hearth-healthy produce shouldn't be hard to find.

Production Enhancing Drugs

Another major source of questionable chemicals is animal products. Fifty years ago, a dairy cow produced 2,000 pounds of milk per year. Today, the average cow gives 50,000 pounds of milk per year. How is such a radical increase possible? Only with the assistance of hormones.

You may think that milk is just milk, but the FDA allows milk producers to give their cows up to eighty-two different drugs, and these never make it onto the Nutrition Facts label. The milk you drink is swimming in hormones. Two of the most-used—bovine growth hormone and estrogen are believed to work together to provoke heart disease.

Cows bred for slaughter are also injected with growth hormones so they grow bigger, faster. Meat has been known to contain up to fourteen times the amount of pesticides and other chemicals as plant foods.[9]

At health food supermarkets you can choose from a variety of milks and meats that are produced without hormones. I encourage you to buy and enjoy the pure stuff to enhance your heart health.

What's In A Name?

One of the biggest jokes the food industry plays is that "lite" and "low-fat" foods are good for you. Nothing could be further from the truth! These labels typically mean the product has less fat than the regular version. I have seen "lite" candy bars and even "lite" Twinkies! You've got to be kidding me!

But harmful chemicals, preservatives and food colorings remain in the foods, along with large amounts of refined sugar, refined flour and processed oils. Nothing healthy has been added. Lately the push is on to produce fake fats, which are essentially plastics, that decrease the calories people absorb from fat. Nabisco launched a product with the texture of fat, "salatrim", for its cookies. The Nutra-Sweet company put imitation ice creams and sherbets on the market but because their texture was not pleasing to the palate, they stopped producing them. A synthetic fat is used in some frozen desserts, and in some cheeses and mayonnaise.

A few years ago the FDA allowed Procter & Gamble to try out a fake fat called Olestra. It passes through the digestive tract without being digested or absorbed, much like gum does when swallowed. The company put it in several products, including potato chips. Olestra caused diahrrea in some people and stomach cramps in others.

But a greater concern with fake fats is that some day they will be found to have harmful long-term effects. Common sense tells us that there are no foods without consequences. Nutritious foods have healthy consequences. Non-nutritious foods have harmful consequences. Either they leave a residue of strange chemicals in our bodies, or they block our intestines from absorbing good things. I am reminded that for many years the medical industry said that cigarettes were healthy. What will they say about these fake fats, processed foods, and hormone-rich meat in twenty years?

The "lite" and "low-fat" labels should be looked on with skepticism. After all, if these foods were helping us be healthier, why are people still getting fatter and why is the incidence of heart disease rising?

"Natural" Food

If we are going to follow the dietary wisdom that has existed for thousands of years, we need to eat foods that have not been manipulated. The best diet is one in which the food is not laden with chemicals, drugs, or hormones; and one in which food is not precooked, processed, genetically altered, frozen, or packaged. Go for fresh, fragrant, bursting-with-flavor foods that were recently harvested, slaughtered, or milked. You will notice a dramatic difference in flavor and your heart will be free of strange or questionable chemicals that could harden your arteries.

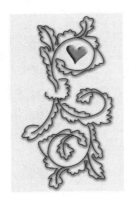

CHAPTER 5
Take A Load Off

The United States of America is one of the largest markets for food items. When I say "largest," I mean it in all senses of the word. This is such an important chapter that I want you to read it without getting defensive. Why do I think that the subject may touch a nerve? It might because more than half of the U.S. population is overweight according to surveys. In fact, they are not just fat; they are excessively fat. This may mean you. Forty-four states of the fifty report dangerously obese populations!

"As obesity rates continue to grow at epidemic proportions in this country, the net effect will be dramatic increases in related chronic health conditions such as diabetes and cardiovascular disease in the future," said a doctor with the Centers for Disease Control and Prevention.[1]   This statement is true but it leads you to believe that the problems will be in the future. The problem is now with over 1.5 million Americans dying of heart disease per year. Most of the heart disease is related to obesity, lack of exercise and smoking.

I am not going to pull any punches as I lay this information out to you. It is vital for you to absorb what I share and put it into action. I will try to be more tactful however than the doctor that was talking with his patient. He said, "Miss, your health problem is that you are fat." The woman, offended, exclaimed, "I want another opinion!" The doctor replied, "Ok, you are ugly too!" Not politically correct but many of my patients' physical ailments have a lot to do with excess weight.

More Is Better

We are living in a society where more is better. Superstores have revolutionized our economy and our lifestyles. Why anybody needs to buy a gallon of honey, a case of Coca-Cola and a twin pack of family sized sugar coated cereals is beyond me; but we do. I think the comedian Louis Andersen explains it best in one of his comedy bits when he talks about going into a mini-mart for a soda. He tells of how the clerk asks, "Do you want the 20 ounce size or the 50 gallon drum?" To which he asks, "What's the difference in price?" "A nickel," answers the clerk. So there goes Louis walking out of the store with the 50 gallon drum and when people give him dirty looks he defends himself screaming, "Hey, it only cost a nickel more! What would you have done?" So true.

Restaurant prices have gone up but in a way, you don't feel so bad because they serve you huge portions. What they serve one person is really enough for two or three but for social pressures, many of us order one plate per person instead of sharing. And a lot of people feel obligated to clean their plates and not let anything go to waste. What about the super size strategies? How many times have you heard, "Would you like to upgrade your fries and soda to extra large for just thirty cents more?" The market is telling us that more is better and we are buying it.

I heard Paul Harvey report that there was a man banned from all of the all-you-can-eat restaurants in a small town because this man would eat all of the food in the entire place. In one case, it was reported that when he finished off the food on the bar, he actually went back into the kitchen and began to cook up more food himself. Wow!

39

We love our food but we are a nation in denial. A report from the Center for Cardiovascular Education stated that most Americans won't admit they have a problem with their weight.[2] Hello! When Yankee Stadium was remodeled, they had to decrease the seating capacity to put in wider seats to fit the fans' fannies. Big is beautiful and people are pleasantly plump. But, all of this wonderful self-esteem boosting is not helping people live longer. The popular thing is to accept yourself, love yourself and your body. OK. Love yourself and your body and shed those pounds so that you will have more energy, feel better and live longer!

More than ten years ago, the Surgeon General warned "for most of us the problem has become one of overeating—too many calories for our activity levels and an imbalance in the nutrients consumed along with them."[3] That really gets to the crux of the problem. We are consuming too many calories and we are doing nothing to burn them off. We are no longer couch potatoes. We are couch potato patches.

Modern society is working against us. We want everything to be convenient. We don't want to move our bodies for anything. Most jobs now are desk jobs. You don't have to get up to change the channel on the television nor to answer the phone. You don't even have to leave the house to go grocery shopping. Just order the groceries online and they will be delivered and let's not even talk about the millions of pizzas delivered to homes across America everyday. When taking a new roll of fax paper to install in the fax machine is considered heavy lifting and golf is considered a physical sport, you just know that society as a whole is not burning off the excess calories.

Obesity generates $68 billion dollars in health care costs per year in the U.S. not counting the $30 billion dollars that Americans spend on weight loss products and services. But as long as people keep ordering their diet sodas to go along with the mega burger, they will not lose weight. You have to control what you

40

eat and do physical activity to burn calories. If you don't, your heart will pay the price.

Weighing On Your Heart

The consequences of being overweight are heavy according to scientific studies. Consider the following:

- Obesity is linked to more than 300,000 premature deaths each year in the U. S., second only to tobacco-related deaths.[4] Studies have found that excess body weight increases the risk of death from heart disease and virtually every other ailment.[5]
- Overweight men and women have a 50 to 72 percent greater chance of a heart attack than non-overweight people.[6]

Are You Overweight?

How do you know if you are overweight? With some people it is obvious but there are others that don't look heavy yet they are overweight. Here is a good indicator. If you are a man and your waist is over 40 inches or if you are a women and your waist is over 35 inches in circumference, your risk for heart disease is higher than other people.[7] I bet you thought I was going to say that you are fat. Forget about being fat or thin, think about the health of your heart.

Here is an important step you can take to determine whether you are overweight or not. Calculate your Body Mass Index (BMI). It is one thing for a six foot tall person to weigh 200 pounds and quite another for a five foot tall person to weigh 200 pounds. BMI is the way to figure out if you are overweight for your height. People with a BMI from 18.5 to around 25 are considered healthy. People with a BMI between 25 and 30 are considered overweight and at moderate risk for heart problems. People with a BMI over 30 are considered to be at high risk.

Let's figure your BMI out right now. Take your weight wearing light clothing and no shoes. Measure your height to the near-

41

est quarter inch. Get your calculator out. Multiply your weight by 705 (don't ask why—it's just part of the formula). If you weigh 155 pounds you would do this:

155 x 705 = 109,275

Don't panic! That's not your BMI! Take that number and divide it by your height in inches. If you are 65 inches tall, your equation would look like this:

109,275 divided by 65 = approx. 1681

Now take that number and divide it by your height one more time. Here is the math using our example:

1681 divided by 65 = 25.86

That is your BMI. In our example, the person is borderline and should probably knock off a few pounds.

Let's do the exercise using my real height and weight. Yikes! I am 69 inches tall and I weigh 170 pounds. Here we go.

170 X 705 = 119,850
119,850/69 = 1,736.9565
1,736.9565/69 = 25.17

Well, I thought it might be worse because I have been a bit chubby since I was a kid but I am not upset because it looks like I am doing pretty good for being 50 years old. Seeing that my BMI is a bit over 25, I know that I am a bit more at risk for a heart problem so I am motivated to keep on going to my spinning classes at the gym. I am including the BMI formula and choles-terol formula in the appendixes at the end of the book for you to fill in. You can also log on to www.nutritionfacts.com to have your

BMI calculated automatically. Please do that and take action accordingly.[8]

Another important point is how your weight is distributed. For women, weight on the thighs and hips is less risky than weight around the waist.[9]

Put plainly, people with pear-shaped bodies, with the bulk of the weight at or below the waistline, are at less risk than people with apple-shaped bodies, where the weight is carried between the neck and waist.[10] If you tend to have an apple shape, you should take the threat of heart disease very seriously and work to get your BMI into an acceptable range.

Like Father Like Son

Be careful with the habits that you are passing on to your kids. Would you believe me if I told you that 70 percent of 12-years-old already have fatty deposits in their arteries?[11]

The Bogalusa Heart Study, the longest and most detailed study of children in the world, found that the major signs of heart disease can be detected in children as young as five years old. Another study found damage in the hearts of subjects as young as three years old.[12] That is remarkable and frightening. Autopsy studies on children have shown lesions in the aorta, coronary vessels and kidney, indicating hard arteries and high blood pressure.[13]

Once again, obesity is the culprit. I don't wonder why either. Have you taken a look at children's menus at restaurants lately? No matter where you go, they are all the same. They offer cheeseburgers, fried chicken fingers, pizza and corndogs. As many as one in four children between the ages of six and seventeen is overweight.[14]

You rarely hear of a child dying from a heart attack but obese children grow up to be at-risk adults. People who were fat as children have a much greater chance of having heart attacks than adults who were not obese as children. Heart trouble can even be predicted by the body shape—apple or pear—of children as young as nine-years-old.[15]

On the other hand, children who jog or play sports are more likely to be fit, and less likely to be fat.[16]

Healthy habits in childhood can stop the hardening of arteries.[17]

"Weight control, and encouragement of physical exercise and a prudent diet, if undertaken early in life, may retard the [hardening of the arteries]," wrote one doctor in a major study of heart disease in children.[18]

Maybe you don't want to deprive your child of the joy of junk food but teaching a child to treat his or her body correctly leads to greater health, well-being, energy and stamina.[19]

Take Charge

If you and your family are overweight, don't turn to fad diets, which often help you lose pounds in the short run but offer no long term solutions. Do the following:

- Eat the kinds of foods that will be talked about in the healthy eating chapters.
- Don't overeat. You can get fat by eating too much of the right foods.
- Limit the times and places you allow yourself to eat.
- Don't snack on unhealthy foods.
- Exercise!

CHAPTER 6
Other Culprits

This section of the book is a bit like being taken out behind the shed for a whipping! I know that I was pretty tough about smoking and overeating. Now I am going to cover a few more enemies of your heart and then we will get into the good stuff in the next section of the book.

High Blood Pressure

We live in a high pressure society. You've got to make the sale, you've got to meet the deadline. If you don't you will lose to your competitor. All this stress is contributing to high blood pressure. High blood pressure is one of the leading contributores to heart disease.

What causes high blood pressure? I mentioned stress and we already covered the other main factor, smoking. Some 50 million Americans suffer from high blood pressure but a third of them don't know it. Studies show that a person with high blood pressure can have two times the normal risk of heart disease.[1]

High blood pressure speeds up the process of hardening of the arteries which increases the buildup of fatty deposits.[2]

What is the impact on the heart? The higher the blood pressure is, the harder the heart has to work. The heart may be up to the task initially but after a period of time, the heart grows stiff and weak.[3] This process may take years. It leads to congestive heart failure and heart attacks.

The good news is that high blood pressure is easily detectable and usually controllable.[4] Have your blood pressure checked regularly, don't smoke, eat right and exercise.

Diabetes

Diabetes is another contributor to heart disease. This is a concern because at least 16 million Americans suffer from diabetes, putting them at much greater risk of heart disease than the general population.[5]

In recent years there has been a drop in heart disease in women accept for women who have diabetes. Those who are at least 55 years old and have diabetes are seven times more likely to have heart disease than women without diabetes.[6]

Diabetics also suffer more arteries clogging up after surgery and they are more likely to die after undergoing angioplasty. One researcher stated "[Re-clogging of the arteries] is one of the strongest predictors (of death after angioplasty) in the diabetic population, ... This study indicates that diabetics should be treated differently from the general population."[7]

Did you know that few people actually die of diabetes? Diabetics usually die from a complication with their hearts. Again, diet and exercise are the keys to preventing or controlling diabetes.

Gum Disease

I bet you had no idea that gingivitis had anything to do with your heart health. Well, it does. You need to avoid gum disease or get rid of it and not just so that you won't have bad breath. It is most likely that the link between gum disease and heart disease is the bacteria that cause the periodontal problem.

People with periodontal disease are fro) r rd to more than two times more likely to have heart disease ople who do not have the condition.[8] That is a very strong r)(iship and suggests that bacteria may be a prime culprit in i t damage. "Prevention of periodontal disease will likely reduce your risk of heart disease," says one leading researcher.[9]

Bacteria in the mouth have been shown to make blood very sticky which can cause clots.[10] Periodontal disease has been linked to diabetes, respiratory problems and premature births.[11]

Research indicates that "gum disease may pose the greatest danger to your heart because the disease provides not only the bacteria, but also the conditions and opportunity for the bacteria to get into the blood through bleeding gums."[12]

Let me give you a few tips of what you can do to take care of your gums, thus lower your risk of heart disease. Brush your teeth well and floss. Also, take vitamin C. People who take less than 60 milligrams of vitamin C a day have higher rates of gum disease. Even three centuries ago, sailors would eat limes to prevent bleeding gums.[13]

Finally, if it has been a while since you have gone to your dentist, get in there and do it. He or she will have a lot more information of how you can brush your troubles away.

47

CHAPTER 7
Back To Basics

 Can you imagine living in a day with no airplanes, automobiles, televisions, radios or computers? Can you imagine living, as they did a hundred years ago, under the threat of various diseases, viruses and plagues that would sweep through a community and kill thousands? Today we have so many mind-boggling technologies and medicines to keep sickness at bay and to make life easier. I am thankful for all of the modern marvels. However, when it comes to food, I'm as old-fashioned as they come.

I believe that the best diet on the planet is the one people ate until the twentieth century. The back to basics primitive diet is based on what the land produced, what grew in the garden, what the cow gave in the way of milk, and what the herd gave in the way of fresh meat. That is the direction we should all be moving if we want to live longer.

The primitive diet means eating things close to how they naturally occur. People who eat primitive diets generally do not suffer from heart disease, obesity, or high blood pressure. In fact, they tend to be extremely physically fit.

There was a dentist in the early part of this century who decided to travel the world to fulfill his wanderlust. His name was

Weston Price. Instead of sticking to the well-trod vacation paths in Europe and America he ventured into then-uncivilized places: forests and jungles in Asia.

Price couldn't help his curiosity when he met people from relatively primitive tribes. He studied the people and found that they did not have the problems with degenerative diseases like heart disease and cancer that westernized people did.[1]

Price, being a dentist, counted cavities and found that less than one percent of the people's teeth were decayed. He found some groups in which tooth decay was actually nonexistent. None of these people brushed their teeth or visited dentists.[2]

Price discovered what other researchers have discovered: that people who eat primitive diets not only avoid western diseases like cancer and even gum disease, they also virtually never have heart disease.

When I began studying the primitive diet I realized that here is a way to make lifestyle changes that have been proven over many centuries in many parts of the world to prevent heart disease. It is not a silver bullet, but it is as close as we can come.

For example, among the Kitava, a primitive people in Papua, New Guinea, heart attacks, strokes and chest pain are virtually non-existent. All the adults have low blood pressure and are lean. But when a Kitava person adopts the western diet, his health changes. One middle-aged Kitava man who moved to the city and became a businessman was found to have higher blood pressure and more body fat.[3]

A group of aboriginal Australians virtually recovered from diabetes in five weeks by returning to their traditional diet. And a group of obese Hawaiians lost an average of five pounds each in three weeks eating their traditional foods in whatever quantity they wanted, and without exercising![4]

In China, a study showed that Chinese people who shift to a western diet increase their risk of heart disease and stroke whereas villagers in rural Chinese villages have the lowest rates of heart disease in the world. The typical village diet consists of very little meat, steamed rice, vegetables and steamed fish or tofu. The incidence of heart disease is incredibly low.

By contrast, the Chinese who live in the modern cities eat much more meat, dairy products and ice cream and have higher rates of heart disease.[5] These are just a few examples, but they make it clear: Eating the types of foods we will look at in the next few chapters can actually keep heart disease at bay.

The Mediterranean Diet

There is a somewhat popular diet that is a throwback to the primitive diets we should be pursuing. The Mediterranean Diet has received a lot of attention in recent years, and for good reason. Many of the changes we need to make are accomplished in this diet. Yet, there is some confusion regarding the definition of the Mediterranean Diet.

Recall the last time you visited an Italian restaurant. As you waited for your meal you probably munched on buttered bread while watching the waiter go by with trays of pasta drenched with cream sauces, meat sauces, and cheese. That is a far cry from what real Mediterranean food is. Real Italians eat pasta with very little meat. They use meat and cheese sparingly, the way Americans use relish. In its essence, the typical Mediterranean diet is the closest thing the western world has to a primitive diet—and it has wide-ranging health benefits.

But in Italian restaurants all over the U.S., dishes are loaded down with fatty sauces and meats. Standard restaurant dishes like fettuccine Alfredo are often laden with as much saturated fat as three pints of butter-almond ice cream! And fried calamari may have as much cholesterol as a four-egg omelet![6]

The traditional Mediterranean diet has eight components: 1) high monounsaturated/ saturated fat ratio, principally from olive oil, 2) moderate alcohol consumption, principally from red wine and almost always during meals, 3) high consumption of legumes,

4) high consumption of whole grains and cereals, including bread, 5) high consumption of fruits, 6) high consumption of vegetables, 7) low consumption of meat and meat products, and 8) moderate consumption of milk and dairy products.[7]

Health care for many of Mediterranean populations was inferior to that available to people in northern Europe and U.S. However, death rates in the Mediterranean region, were generally lower and adult life expectancy generally higher compared with the more economically developed countries of the north of Europe and North America, particularly among men.[8] A dramatic lower incidence of myocardial infarction and death was reported in patients consuming the Mediterranean-type diet.

The real Mediterranean diet is very healthy and is associated with low risk of heart disease. The usual ingredients are fresh fish, steamed vegetables, olive oil, red wine, and fresh fruit. If you stick with these basic foods, you will be eating the time-honored primitive diet and your heart will fall in love with you all over again.

A Change of Heart

Making the changes I am recommending, like buying fresh and organic foods and avoiding processed foods, may seem difficult, but it is the only sensible way to gain greater heart health. Some day, perhaps not long from now, eating chemically processed, nutritionally empty food will be declared a health hazard, and most of the things that stock the shelves of grocery stores will be a thing of the past. Until then, be aggressive with your health and your diet. Set the pace for healthy living and your heart will reward you with a long and active life.

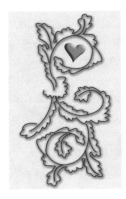

CHAPTER 8
A Healthy Appetite

The National Obsession

Americans have a fascination with food. We eat more than just about every other nation in the world. I remember asking a group of high school students returning from Europe what they thought of the food there. Their response surprised me. "They eat like birds," one young man said disdainfully.

I smiled on the inside because it had not occured to this teenage boy with a bottomless stomach that, in fact, Europeans do not eat like birds. It would be more accurate to say that Americans eat like pigs. A Saturday afternoon trip to Claim Jumpers restaurant and a glance at the portions there should be enough to convince even the staunchest skeptic that Americans wolf down a lot of grub. Food is an integral part of every American's personal history and cultural heritage. Ask any American teenager if they can remember the first time they had a Krispy Kreme donut and you will get an answer.

Americans share a great deal of food experience. Most Americans have sucked the inside out of a Twinkie, twisted the halves of an Oreo cookie apart and scraped off the filling with the lower teeth, and plucked pepperoni slices off a pizza. Food sustains us, and it can be a source of considerable pleasure. It is a reflection of our rich social fabric. It brings families together and becomes part of our fondest memories. And so, when anyone attempts to impose restrictions on this most coveted of pleasures, resistance is inevitable. We seem to think it is our right to eat whatever we want, whenever we want, without consequences. Yet, what we eat is one of the most significant keys for preventing and reversing heart disease.

We Digest With the Heart

People have known for a long time that there was a connection between diet and the health of the heart. Believe it or not, the Bible even mentions it. Yet, the modern medical community rejected the idea that diet caused heart disease until very recently. It took skeptical scientists and doctors decades of research to affirm that diet could cause or prevent disease. Finally, in 1989, the assistant secretary for health wrote:

> Diseases such as coronary heart disease, stroke, cancer and diabetes remain leading causes of death and disability in the United States. Substantial scientific research over the past few decades indicates that diet can play an important role in prevention of such conditions.[1]

The report went on to say that heart disease was linked to unbalanced diets,[2] and that a reduction in the intake of fat and other foods should reduce the risk of heart disease.[3] At the close of the preface, the assistant secretary for health wrote:

> This report ends any scientific controversy. There is no doubt that diet affects chronic-disease risk. In addition, because of the enormity of the impact of diet-related diseases, the report demonstrates that virtually all Americans will benefit from following these recommendations.

Even though the results of various individual studies may be inconclusive, the preponderance of the evidence presented in the Report's comprehensive scientific review substantiates an association between dietary factors and rates of chronic diseases.[4]

The foods we eat are the single most important factor in determining whether or not we develop heart disease. Few would contest

53

that changing our diets would vastly improve our health and reduce a great deal of needless suffering on a worldwide level. Improving diet appears to be a universally accepted goal, but the good intentions of the mainstream medical community have been undercut by a lack of focus and the distractions of the marketplace.

First, the mainstream medical community has targeted cholesterol and fat intake as the most important factors in the prevention of heart disease. While these are important factors in the development of heart disease, they are certainly not the primary culprits. Yet, the public has been led to believe otherwise.

The marketplace has muddied the waters even more. While doctors work to educate us against dietary evils the food industry continues to develop "healthy" foods that do not improve our health at all. Fake fats, non-calorie sweeteners and other such wonders have given us little more than the false confidence that we are getting healthier when the opposite is true.

The government's attempts to educate people about food is commendable. However, the government's policy to protect the food industry is appalling. Chemical manipulation of foods to increase productivity, shelf-life and economic gain contribute to the very explosion of the diseases we want to prevent. Yet, these industry processes are protected by the federal government.

Where can a conscientious public turn for guidance? Increasingly, doctors are telling their patients to reconsider high carbohydrate/low-fat diet recommended by the American Heart Association. According to Dr. Michael Eades, many researchers and physicians are "quickly moving in this direction." He adds that, "organizations like the American Diabetes Association are trying to save face by *slowly* changing their focus." Unfortunately, many people embrace the advice of popular diet "experts."

There are many recommended diets in circulation today. Some experts promote diets high in proteins, some promote diets high in carbohydrates are the cure, some promote diets composed exclusively of fruits and vegetables. High-profile doctors like Atkins and Ornish will vigorously defend their theories for a universal diet. All experts claim to possess irrefutable scientific evidence in support of their theories.

Whose expert advice should we follow? Atkins and Ornish practically came to blows in a heated debate over their respective diets at a conference I attended in Orlando not too long ago. Both best-selling authors regaled each other with evidence and testimonials. I'm sure their debate convinced some in attendance, but I'm guessing that a good deal of people left more confused than ever. What we desperately need is practical, unbiased, unrestricted, non-discriminative, universal dietary wisdom.

Don't misunderstand me. I am not going to propose a new diet. Remember, I am in favor of a primative diet.

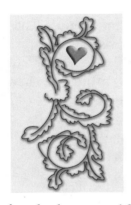

CHAPTER 9
Eat To The Beat Of A Different Drum

A Little of This and a Little of That

Hippocrates said that you enjoy health only if you and your body are in perfect balance with the environment. Eating habits have become severely unbalanced in the past two hundred years and fat consumption has increased dramatically since the nineteenth century from about 20% of a person's energy intake to about 50% today. This has happened despite the fact that people today need much less energy, given that we are far less physically active.[1] During the same period of time, the amounts of fresh fruits, vegetables, nuts, and whole grains we eat have shrunk to half the amount people used to eat. People are not getting nearly as many vitamins, phytonutrients, antioxidants, and other important substances found in these foods.

The average person consumes approximately sixty tons of food in a lifetime. That's like eating everything in the grocery store. Everything. With what will you stock the aisles of your personal grocery store? The universal dietary "laws" I propose are as old as the Bible, one of the oldest known records of lifestyle recommendations. The general principles of this diet can keep our hearts healthier than anything on the market today.

The dietary wisdom that we are about to explore is, after more than 4000 years, up-to date and validated by modern scientific methodology. These guidelines apply to you regardless of your preference for meats or vegetables, your emotional type, your blood type, your ethnic background, your age, your sex,etc. This dietary wisdom is universal, and if you follow it, you will drastically reduce your chances of heart disease.

Fruits and Vegetables
Without reservation I make the following statement to the general public. The best thing we can do for the heart from a dietary point of view is to eat more fruits and vegetables. If you are going to choose to incorportate only one new habit into your regular dietary practices, you would be wise to choose this one. Without question fruits and vegetables are the backbone of any heart-healthy diet.

Modern science backs up what many cultures have know for thousands of years. Studies show time and again that people who eat a lot of fruits and vegetables have a reduced risk of heart disease.[2] A study in Finland during the early 1970s showed that people began eating substantially more fruit and vegetables and that the dietary trend coincided with a decline in death from heart disease.[3] Even the famous Dr. Ornish found that people in his study who ate vegetarian diets had half the number of heart problems as people who ate the typical American diet.[4]

Fruits and vegetables don't contain cholesterol, and they are naturally low in saturated fat, calories, and sodium. They are also rich in protein, potassium, fiber, folic acid, and vitamin C. Numerous studies have been conducted showing the health benefits derived from the regular consumption of fruits and vegetables. A study in Italy showed that high vegetable consumption decreased heart attacks dramatically.[5] Another study showed that a diet high in fruits, vegetables, and nuts actually lowers a person's blood pressure.[6]

There are a number of substances present in most fruits and vegetables that assist the body in the prevention of heart disease. One set of these substances are called phytochemicals. The first of these phytochemicals are the sterols. *Sterols* appear to block cholesterol absorption from dietary intake. In other words, they keep our bodies from soaking up large amounts of harmful cholesterols from the foods we eat. Think of the salad you eat before the steak is served as a small measure of prevention. These sterols also increase cholesterol excretion from the body. So, not only do they keep cholesterols from getting inside the body, but they also round up excess cholesterol already present in our systems and escort it out.[7] Want a salad with that meal?

The second of these phytochemicals are called flavonoids. *Flavonoids* prevent LDL cholesterol oxidation, thus delaying the development of hard arteries.[8] Flavonoid intake has been shown to reduce the fatality rates from heart disease and the incidence of heart attack. In the Zutphen Elderly Study, elderly men with the highest consumption of flavonoids over a five-year period had 60 percent less mortality from heart disease than low flavonoid consumers.[9]

The last of these essential phytochemicals are sulfur compounds. *Sulfur Compounds* are found in the allium family of vegetables, which includes garlic, onions and leeks. It has been shown that garlic possesses preventive and protective properties against cardiovascular disease.[10] The point I want to make to you is that virtually every fruit and vegetable you can think of possesses a substance that will present a health benefit to your heart. Find fruits and vegetables that you enjoy eating and start buying them every week. If you are worried about variety . . . don't. Nobody ever died from eating only apples and carrots during the apple and carrot season and ignoring oranges and celery. You will still derive tremendous benefit from regular consumption of whatever fruits and vegetables happen to be in season.

Phytochemicals are not the only substances present in fruits and vegetables that fight heart disease. The pigments that provide color to fruits and vegetables also protect us from heart disease. The reddish pigments found in strawberries, cherries, raspberries, cranberries, blueberries, grapes, and black currants provide protection against heart disease by slowing the generation of cholesterol. Remember, most of the cholesterol present in the body is produced by the body. If we want to lower our cholesterol level, what better way than to eat foods that will regulate the internal factory that produces cholesterol, the liver.[11]

There are some benefits that are exclusive to vegetables. For example, eating veggies helps the body balance blood sugar levels. A study conducted in Britain found that people who ate salad and raw vegetables frequently year-round had an over 80 percent lower risk of adult-onset diabetes than people who ate vegetables less often. This is only scratching the surface. The reality is that there are hundreds of benefits to be derived from eating these foods and each individual fruit or vegetable often presents its own unique health benefit. Without question, the evidence is overwhelmingly in favor of eating a good deal of fruits and vegetables. So, how much is a good deal, exactly?

Most nutritionists recommend eating five servings of fruits and vegetables every day. Yet, drive by a fast food restaurant during the lunch hour and you will see a line of cars at the drive up window. I can guarantee you that a quick trip past the fruit stand will not reveal a similar line of cars. I am sad to report that the average American eats fewer than two servings of vegetables per day and less than one serving of fruit. This is astonishing considering the fact that we are so pressed for time. After all, fruits and vegetables are the ultimate fast food. Wash an apple and eat it, peel a banana and eat it, grab a handful of carrot sticks and eat them. There is no excuse for not eating enough of these foods.

If you love your heart, you will decide right now to add more fruits and vegetables to your diet. If you already eat plenty of them, I applaud you. If not, make it a habit. Buy apples instead of potato chips, oranges instead of candy bars, and stock your fridge and fruit bowl with bananas, pears, or whatever else is in season. Bring a bag of celery sticks and carrots to work with you. Next time you're in a restaurant, order a salad instead of an appetizer of deep-fried mozzerella sticks.

Recognizing the availability of these foods will make all the difference in the world. After just a few days or weeks your body will begin to crave these foods like you used to crave unhealthy foods. Again, I will say there is no better way to prevent heart disease than to add more fruits and vegetables to your diet.

Downsizing

While there are many foods that we should incorporate into our diet, there are some things we should cut out of our diet, too. We can not expect to dramatically improve our health and life expectancy without some measure of sacrifice. After increasing the consumption of fruits and vegetables, reducing our animal fat consumption is the second most important dietary correction we can make.

Fat is a major culprit in the development of heart disease, but it depends on the kind of fat and how much is consumed. Animal fats are among the worst for our hearts. Recent findings from the Oxford Vegetarian Study show that vegetarians had a 39 percent lower death rate due to heart disease than people who eat meat at least once a week. Fish eaters showed similar results as vegetarians. There is a strong correlation between higher consumption of animal fats and the risk of death by heart disease.[12] The highest coronary heart disease mortality rates in the world are in Eastern block countries in which lard and beef tallow are cornerstones of the diet.[13]

While it appears that animal fats are harmful, it is equally evident that other fats are not, if eaten in moderation.[14] Other fats, like those from olive and canola oils, are healthier. Recent studies have shown that the fat in these oils, bring down plasma cholesterol levels.[15]

60

Unfortunately, about 50 percent of the saturated fat and 70 percent of the cholesterol in our diet comes from hamburgers, cheeseburgers, meat loaf, beef steaks, roasts, hot dogs, ham, lunch meat, doughnuts, cookies, cakes, whole milk, cheese, ice cream, and eggs. To reduce the risk of coronary heart disease, people should restrict their intake of these foods and eat poultry (white meat without the skin), fish, skimmed or low-fat milk, nonfat or low-fat yogurt and low-fat cheeses. Unsaturated vegetable oils such as soybean, corn, olive, and canola are also good, but should be eaten in moderation because they are high in calories. Consumption of foods rich in hydrogenated vegetable oils like margarine, cookies, and french fries should be avoided.

But let's not fall into the trap of excluding all fat from our diet. The key is moderation. By cutting back our consumption of animal fats and non-naturally occurring fats, we will experience significant improvement in our chances of developing heart disease.

A heart can beat forever under ideal conditions. Unfortunately we live in a world that presents us with less than ideal conditions. While nobody can live forever, it is within your power and mine to lengthen our lives. I believe that even people who only take these two steps will see an improvement in their overall health and a reduction in their risk of developing heart disease.

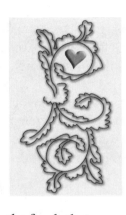

CHAPTER 10
A Real Meal Deal

Food as Armor
While the addition of fruits and vegetables and the reduction of saturated fat intake are the most important dietary adjustments we can make, there are other foods that defend the body from heart disease. Many of the foods that possess these hidden benefits may surprise you.

Oil the Pump
Olive oil is a really important food that has been a staple element of healthy diets for thousands of years. This oil possesses many healthful attributes. Modern science has been quick to recognize the benefits this product brings to the heart.

Olive oil is one of the healthiest oils on the planet. These Mediterranean plants experience long exposure to sunlight, thus increasing the levels of a substance called phenols in the olives. The phenols in olive oil inhibit the oxidation of LDL cholesterol. Therefore, when we eat olive oil consistantly, our arteries will experience less damage over that time.[1] Italian scientists recently reported that patients with high blood pressure reduced the amount of blood pressure-lowering drugs they needed by switching to a diet low in saturated fat and rich in olive oil. What's more, some of the patients were able to stop their high blood pressure medication completely with the dietary changes. The phenols in olive oil are responsible for reducing the need of blood pressure medication because they stimulate the production of substances that increase the opening of arteries, which in turn reduces artery resistance to blood flow, and as a result blood pressure is decreased.[2]

Olive oil is a delicious cooking aid and works well as a substitute for butter or margarine. Instead of putting a stick of butter on the table, put a bowl of oil and dip warm bread into it. You and your family will discover what the Italians, Greeks, and French have known about for centuries and your heart will be healthier.

The Nuts and Bolts of Health

I don't know about you, but my idea of a great Monday evening involves sitting in front of the television watching the football game with a bowl of mixed nuts in a bowl on my lap. I like them all; almonds, walnuts, cashews, pecans, etc. You name it, I'll eat it. I know what you are thinking. Traditionally, nuts have been off limits to people on diets because of the high fat content. It is true that about 60 percent of the weight and 80 percent of the calories in most nuts come from fat.

Yet, nuts have been a common element in the diets of healthy people for centuries. There is a reason for that. Modern research provides an explanation. In five of the best and largest studies on heart disease report that eating nuts frequently is associated with a decreased risk of heart disease. In fact, no other food has been so consistently associated with a marked reduction in heart disease risk in people of all habits, races and health profiles.[3]

Those who eat lots of nuts experience an extra five years of life expectancy free of heart disease and an 18 percent lifetime risk of heart disease compared with 30 percent in people who eat few nuts.[4] A 50-gram serving of nuts exceeds the recommended daily allowance for vitamin E, which has been shown to reduce the risk of coronary heart disease.[5]

You would do well to incorporate nuts into your daily life, whether that means including them in your recipes or keeping a bowl of them on the table. It is true that dry roasted nuts, which are often heavily salted, are not as healthy for you as those that are less processed. However, if flavor is an issue for you, simply mix the two together in a bowl. For the health-conscious person, nuts are no longer taboo.

Fruit of the Vine

If you ever get the oppotunity to tour the wine country of California by hot-air balloon, seize the chance. You will never forget the stunning beauty of the vineyards and surrounding countryside. Not only is it an absolutely breath-taking experience, but you gain a bird's eye view of one of the most widely consumed fruits in the world. Grapes are not only one of the world's most popular fruits, but they also possess wonderfully heart-healthy attributes. Grapes, too, have been a regular dietary component of many healthy cultures for centuries.

Again, modern scientific research explains the benefits of consuming grapes. In a very recent study, researchers found that drinking an average of two cups of purple grape juice a day for one week vastly reduced the "stickiness" of blood platelets. This is good news for those wanting to prevent heart disease. When the blood is sticky there is a greater chance of the development of arteriosclerosis, the primary cause of heart disease. By comparison, other juices like orange juice and grapefruit juice showed no such effect.

The difference may be due to the different kinds of substances they contain. Purple grape juice has approximately three times the polyphenols of citrus juices. Polyphenols are powerful agents in the war against heart disease.[6] Grape juice also appears to contribute to the opening of the arteries. Therefore, the combination of these two effects decreases the risk of blood clots and heart attack.[7]

64

Eating our fill of grapes would do most of us a world of good. Every school child who brought their lunch to school in a brown paper bag knows how good a cluster of grapes can taste in the middle of the day. Crisp and refreshing, they burst with flavor and life. Take a bunch of grapes to work instead of waiting for the afternoon break to buy a candy bar from the vending machine. Consider replacing soda and sugary-sweet drinks with refreshing grape juice. Again, availability of this healthy drink in your refrigerator will make the difference. This small change may help to save your life.

One Glass a Day Keeps the Doctor Away

In recent years, a remarkably consistent body of evidence has been collected suggesting that those who drink alcohol moderately have a reduced risk of coronary heart disease compared to those who abstain from alcohol. This preventive effect of alcohol may be largely confined to the middle-aged and older.[8] In contrast, binge drinking, a practice engaged in particularly by young men, and chronic heavy drinking can negate the heart-healthy benefits of alcohol. Instead, such patterns of drinking increase the risk of hypertension, stroke, heart attack, and heart disease in general.[9]

Alcoholic beverages have been in existence for thousands of years, albeit in far less potent forms. Historically, many cultures have not looked down on moderate consumption and have still experienced considerable longevity. Therefore, the rule is quite easy to follow. Less than two drinks per day of any kind of alcohol is associated with a 50 percent reduction in the risk of heart disease. At the same time, more than two drinks per day increases the risk of heart disease, heart attack, and stroke 100 to 200 percent.[10] How is it that a trip to the pub or a glass of wine at dinner is good for us?

There are several credible theories about why alcohol reduces heart disease. At least half of the protective action appears to be explained by the increase in HDL cholesterol levels that

65

occur after consumption. This increase often improves the ratio of HDL cholesterol to LDL cholesterol. Remember, cholesterol ratios are more important than total level.

In addition, alcohol also keeps blood platelets from sticking and piling up on artery walls. This helps to prevent atherosclerosis, which is the primary cause of heart disease, stroke, and heart attack. A glass of wine will lubricate the blood, if you will.

All of this poses a dilemma from a public health standpoint, and from a religious standpoint. If a person is morally opposed to drinking alcohol, how do they incorporate this knowledge into their lifestyles, or do they? Personally, I recommend that the individual consult their own conscience. The benefits of drinking alcohol are not significant enough to go against one's morals, and most of the beneficial effects of alcohol can be achieved by a low-fat diet alone. But the heart does seem to benefit from moderate alcohol consumption, red wine in particular.

Health in a Bottle
By far the most popular and the healthiest alcoholic drink is red wine. Red wine contains abundant polyphenols. These antioxidants offer a series of benefits to our cardiovascular system. For one, red wine has been shown to inhibit LDL cholesterol oxidation. This helps to prevent atherosclerosis. Red wine also increases antioxidant capacity and raises the levels of HDL cholesterol. Needless to say, all of these things are necessary elements in an effective battle against heart disease.[11]

Red wine might help explain the "French paradox." For years, scientists were baffled by the low incidence of heart disease mortality in France despite the high incidence of risk factors such as smoking, a high-fat diet and lack of exercise among the French. In fact, the French enjoy the lowest incidence of heart disease mortality of all industrialized nations.[12] Now we suspect that it is the glass of red wine, a staple at the dinner table in France, that is responsible for this anomaly.

Drinking two servings of red wine per day will provide approximately 40 percent of the total antioxidant polyphenols present in a healthy diet, as well as polyphenols that are virtually absent from fruit and vegetables. Wine holds an advantage over vegetables in that its polyphenols are much more easily absorbed by the body. The only other substance that enjoys such an advantage is tea.

Its in the Leaves

Ask the average teenager what the most popular drink in the world is and they will say Pepsi Twist. Ask a college student and they will say beer. Of course the correct answer is water, but what you may not know is that tea runs right behind in second place. In fact, it has for a long, long time. You also may be unaware of the tremendous benefits tea offers the heart.

Scientist have found that up to fifty percent of the extractable solids of green tea leaves are polyphenolic compounds. Polyphenols are antioxidants, which are powerful agents in the fight against heart disease. A single cup of green tea usually contains about 200–400 mg of polyphenols. Green teas show heavier antioxidant concentrations than the black teas more common in America. Studies have indicated that drinking tea protects against heart disease.[13] Hey! Fifty million Chinese can't be wrong.

A Cup of Joe to Go, Please

Americans are caffeine addicts. No question. Everytime it rains in the continental U.S. a Starbucks coffee shop sprouts up out of the ground. I'm joking, of course, but not really. When you walk into the office today, count how many people you see clutching a hot cup of coffee. They will not be in the minority I can assure you.

Coffee has gotten a bad rap in recent years. Yet, it has been around for a long time. It is not that the accusations were unsubstantiated. For almost 70 years we've recognized that moderate doses of caffeine elevates blood pressure. Coffee consumption has been associated with an increased risk of stroke for men with high blood pressure over the age of 55. The risk was more than doubled for men who consumed three cups of coffee per day compared to those who did not drink coffee.[14]

Yet, despite the general impression that high coffee consumption is bad, the Scottish Heart Study found the prevalence of heart disease to be the highest among those who abstain from coffee drinking and lowest among those who drink five or more cups per day in Scotland.[15] Therefore, the jury is still out on this one. My recommendation is to limit consumption to less than two cups a day. Whatever your coffee habits are, some restriction of regular coffee intake may be beneficial, particularly for older individuals with high blood pressure.

You're Not Going to Believe This But . . .

Chocolate is actually good for you! Can you believe it? After all, it has been a food product of Central and South America for hundreds of years. Of course this does not mean that we should rush out and stock up on Snickers bars, but it does mean we can absolve ourselves from the guilt of eating an occasional candy bar.

Recently it was shown that chocolate contains large amounts of polyphenols that have potent anti-oxidant activities.[16] A small piece of milk chocolate contains almost as many polyphenols as a standard serving of red wine.[17] The polyphenols in chocolate help to prevent hardening of the arteries. Research suggests that dietary intake of chocolate may reduce the risk of atherosclerosis, and mortality from heart disease.

Of course, eating too much chocolate is not recommended. Chocolate is made with large amounts of refined sugar, which is definately not good for you. But if you want an occasional sugary snack, chocolate is a good alternative.

Fiber

Ancient peoples have recognized the health benefits of fiber. Just about every ancient culture produced food products from whole grains. Over the past 20 years, many studies have investigated the association between dietary fiber and risk for coronary heart disease. The evidence strongly suggests that dietary fiber reduces the risk of heart disease.

Virtually every major supermarket in America today offers consumers a choice of whole-grain products to purchase. Whole-grain fiber is extremely good for you and is an essential element to a heart-healthy diet. Clinical trials suggest that the intake of whole-grains like wheat, rice, and oats has the strongest preventive effect on heart disease.[18]

Similar studies revealed that those who ate whole wheat bread had fewer heart attacks than those who ate white bread. The risk was far less for people who ate whole-wheat bread than those who ate white bread because white bread contains very little fiber.[19] Another study among postmenopausal women showed that those who ate more whole grain experienced 33 percent less risk of heart disease death when compared with people who ate little or no whole grain.[20]

Many people are under the assumption that the fruits they eat will provide a sufficient amount of dietary fiber. Understand, there are two kinds of fiber. There are soluble fibers, like fruit fibers, which dissolve in water. There are also non-soluble fibers, like whole-grain fibers, which do not dissolve in water. Soluble fibers decrease LDL cholesterol levels, which may explain their protective role in the prevention of heart disease, but non-soluble fibers offer tremendous benefits too.

From the Nurses' Health Study, it was observed among different sources of dietary fiber, that only consumption of whole-grain fiber was strongly associated with a reduced risk of heart disease. The study showed that women in the group who ate the most whole-grain, which was about 2.5 servings per day, experienced a more than 30 percent lower risk of heart disease than the group who ate little whole-grain. Almost the same results were observed in men in the Health Professionals Follow-up Study.[21]

Unfortunately, when 4,000 American households were sur-
veyed, the results were pitifully unhealthy. The average consumption of whole-grain products is only about 0.5 servings per day
per person.[22] Yet, the Food Guide Pyramid of the U.S. Department of Agriculture recommends six to eleven servings of grain
products per day. Unfortunately, the amount of whole grains is
not specified. Most of the grain products consumed in the U.S.
are highly refined, causing them to lose 99 percent of their fiber.

To get whole-grain products you only need to look for them.
Whole-grain breads, cereals and flour are available in virtually
any grocery store. It's about time you had the best part of the
grain.

Hooked on Oil

Fishing is one of the oldest professions. This is for the obvious
reason that people have long recognized that the lakes, rivers,
and oceans of the world contain an abundant source of food.
Personally, I love seafood. If it lives in the ocean, I will eat it. One
of the things that makes fish so easy to incorporate into a diet is its
versatility. There are so many different ways to prepare and flavor
fish that everyone can find a few recipes that are appealing to the
taste buds.

Fish are also an important food for us to consume if we want
to prevent heart disease. Scientists tell us that fish are a major
source of omega-3 fatty acids, which are important to the human
body. The omega-3 fatty acids from fish protect us against heart
disease and prevent deaths from heart disease and heart attack.[23]

Research reveals exactly how these fatty acids provide protection to us. The unique properties of omega-3 fatty acids first
become apparent when researchers were studying Greenland
Eskimos who consumed diets very high in fat from seals, whales,
and fish and yet had a low rate of heart disease.[24]

Further studies clarified the paradox. The fat that Eskimos
consumed contained large quantities of the omega-3 fatty acids

which are abundant in fish, shellfish, and sea mammals.[25] Research revealed that dietary omega-3 fatty acids reduce heart disease risk by preventing the formation of blood clots, widening the arteries, inhibiting plaque formation, reducing high blood pressure and preventing arteries from becoming inflamed.

Omega-3 fatty acids also increase production of nitric oxide, which relaxes your arteries.[26] Omega-3 fatty acids also seem to behave like aspirin does, acting against inflammation. They reduce the number of white blood cells that respond to inflammation, thereby reducing the risk of chronic inflammation.[27] Wow! Talk about food that packs a wallop.

Some fatty fish, most notably mackerel, herring, salmon and halibut, are rich sources of these fatty acids.[28] In recent years, the recommended level of omega-3 fatty acids in the diet has been debated. There have even been recommendations that would require four-fold increase in fish consumption in the U.S. or the use of fish-oil supplements. I tend to agree that most people should eat much more fish than they currently do.[29]

Certainly, research encourages us to incorporate more fish into our diet. In one study, men who ate salmon more than one time a week had a 70 percent reduction in the risk of primary cardiac arrest.[30] In another study, the total mortality rate was decreased by 29 percent in men with overt cardiovascular disease who derived sufficient amounts of omega-3 fatty acids from fish or fish oil.[31]

In a third study, a diet rich in omega-3 fatty acids was given to a group of heart attack survivors and they experienced a 76 percent decrease in cardiac deaths compared with the group of patients that received a conventional diet.[32] The most recent study on fish consumption showed that consumption of more than one fatty fish meal a week was associated with a 52 percent lower risk of sudden cardiac death compared with consumption of less than one fish meal per month.[33]

The current consensus is that eating fish is beneficial at surprisingly modest intakes, and the benefit probably depends on the fatty acid profile of the fish. There does not appear to be a greater reduction in the risk of heart disease death, especially sudden deaths, in those who ate more than 1–2 fatty fishmeals per week.[34]

People who are unable to eat fish or shellfish can take fish oil supplements. For primary prevention, 2–3 grams of fish oil per day is desirable. Higher doses should be used for prevention of a second heart attack. However, fish is not the only source of these fatty acids.

Plants also provide a rich source of another omega-3 fatty acid. Vegetable oils like canola, cottonseed, and soybean oils are a major source. Other plant sources include nuts, seeds, vegetables, legumes, grains and some fruit. Of these specific foods, nuts, seeds and soybeans are relatively high in omega-3 fatty acids.[35]

Research should encourage us to consume these products as well. Olive, canola, walnut, and flaxseed oil, which all contain omega-3 fatty acid, have been medically proven to lower blood pressure. In one study women with moderately high blood pressure switched to olive oil for a month and had significant drops in blood pressure.[36] The lesson from history and science is simple. Consume foods that contain these fatty acids and you will be taking steps to prevent heart disease.

It takes decades for heart disease to creep up on us, so the food we eat during those years can make a huge difference. Doctors, drugs, and technology may be able to temporarily bail us out after heart disease has set in, but they do not offer a cure. In fact, the best medicine has to offer is a high-tech plumbing job that may or may not buy us more time. By the time you subject yourself to the medical mill of currently fashionable treatments, you have already gambled with the outcome. But proper dietary changes now can keep you healthy without the need for medical interventions, like surgery or drugs.

If more people practiced prevention through diet and other lifestyle habits, life spans would lengthen and heart disease would not be nearly as common as it is today. According to the National

Center for Health Statistics, if all forms of heart disease were eliminated, the average life span would rise by almost ten years. If all forms of cancer were eliminated, the gain would be only three years.

In fact, heart disease should not take any lives at all. I believe the vast majority of deaths due to heart disease were originally preventable. All it would have taken was a change in a few lifestyle habits.

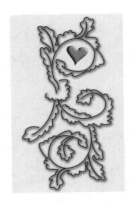

CHAPTER 11
Get A Move On

There is an exercise craze going on right? The gyms are full and everyone is wearing more and more revealing clothes to show off their abdomen's, sleek legs, powerful arms and other parts we don't need to mention. Exercise is big business. The television is full of infomercials selling ab busters this and ab busters that, thigh masters this and buns of steel that. I think two products in particular reflect reality. The first one is the pill that speeds up your metabolism. That way, you burn calories even when you are asleep. The other product is the one that you strap on electrodes that cause your abdomen to contract. Supposedly, you receive the same benefits as you do from doing sit-ups but you don't have to do the work. Though beautiful bodies are paraded before us on television, and we spend tons of money on products to make us look that way, our desire for comfort, convenience and indulgence is greater than our vanity.

The statistics clearly demonstrate that the hard bodies that are truly fit are the minority. If you are like most people, you know that you need to work out but you don't. The most common excuse given for not exercising is, "I can't find the time." That is interesting when you consider that exercising will add years to your life. Let me say that in a different way. If you don't exercise, statistics indicate that your lifespan will be shorter. That is a literal loss of time. So make time to exercise.

Motivation

Getting started is probably the hardest part. Keeping it going is also difficult. You have to find the right motivation to really stick with it. Vanity for some people is all it takes. But for others, we need to find a motivation that is more than skin deep. It takes a complete commitment to get a rock hard supermodel body. But it does not take that much effort to get life extending benefits from exercise. So for me, the motivation factors are that I feel better, I have more energy, I have more endurance and I will add years to my life that I can spend enjoying my children and wife, my future grandchildren and the different projects and ministries that I am involved with. When I exercise, I think about all of those things and it actually becomes a bit of a spiritual experience.

Another thing that really helps is if you can get involved in sports. Playing basketball is a lot of fun and boy does it work you out. I love to play tennis and swim as well. I enjoy playing sports but they also motivate me to get in the gym because I want to be able to keep up with the younger generation and increase my enjoyment. I just love to snow ski but it takes so much strength in the legs to do it well and to make the most of a day out on the slopes. That is another reason that really keeps me going to the gym. I hear so many people complaining that they are always tired. The best advice I can give them is to exercise. There are a number of reasons why exercising boosts your energy.

The Impact of Exercise

Your body benefits in so many ways from exercise. The end results are that you will be more healthy, feel better and have more energy. What goes on in your body when you exercise? This is one of the best ways to clean out the crud in your body.

When you work up a great sweat, your body starts to excrete toxins right through your skin. Sweating is actually a more powerful way to detox your body than urinating! Did you know that our body has a fluid in it that has the responsibility of taking poisons out of our body? We do. It is the lymph. But unlike blood that has a pump (the heart) the lymphatic system does not have a pump. The flow of the lymph is dependent on the movement of the body. So get a move on and start getting poisons out of your body.

Another fantastic fact is that when you exercise, your body releases little chemicals called endorphins that decrease pain and produce a slight feeling of euphoria. That's right, exercise produces a natural high. Putting your body into motion will tone your muscles and increase your strength and endurance. It also relieves emotional stress so it can really help you get through the day.

Direct Benefits For Your Heart
Recently a study concluded that a healthy lifestyle could reduce the probability of heart disease by 82 percent. Not even price slashes at Wal-Mart can offer such a great reduction! This landmark study, called the Nurses' Health Study, was conducted at the Harvard School of Public Health, and was the first to show what happens when people do everything they are supposed to, the same things that are covered in this book —eating right, smoking cessation, weight control, limiting consumption of alcoholic beverages and, yes, you guessed it.......exercise! This study conducted with 84,000 nurses found that those who exercised vigorously for thirty minutes a day in combination with other healthy habits were the ones who lowered their risk of heart attacks, congestive heart failure and stroke.[1] The study reports that these results "are very dramatic because these are not drastic changes for people. Premature heart disease can be virtually eliminated by these lifestyle changes."[2]

Another study showed that men who run the most had lower blood pressure and higher levels of high-density lipoprotein (HDL),

76

which is good cholesterol. Long-term endurance increases longevity by reducing blood pressure, body fat and bad cholesterol.[3]

A Harvard study that followed the lives of 17,300 middle-aged men for more than twenty years found that vigourous activities dramatically reduced the risk of dying, The *Journal of the American Medical Association* reported that men who did at least 1,500 calories' worth of jogging, brisk walking or other vigorous activity each week had a 25 percent lower death rate during the study period than those who expended less than 1,500 calories a week.

The more active the men were, the longer they were likely to live—even the men with bad habits like smoking and drinking. Researchers agreed that exercise increased their longevity because it reduced the risk of heart disease.[4]

You can actually add years to your life by exercising regularly. If you start exercising at age 35, you can add 6.2 months to your life, studies show. Imagine what you could do if you began even earlier![5]

Let me rattle off some more benefits of excercise:
• You don't need a pill to benefit from it.
• You will live longer.
• Your risk of heart disease will decrease.
• It is more effective than drugs for treating depression.
• It lowers blood pressure.
• It lowers body weight.
• It lowers the risk of developing diabetes.
• It lifts spirits.
• It triggers other healthy lifestyle changes like improving our diet or quitting smoking.[6]

I wish I could invent a healthy lifestyle pill. I would call it, "Silver Bullet." Why do I think that it would be a huge success? Because people are always looking for a silver bullet to solve their problems instead of taking responsibility for their health and doing the right things. But if you look for fun ways to live life healthy and you can do it with your spouse or a good friend, you will be so happy that you did. Exercise is wonderful and there is no downside to it. Now that you know all of this information, let me give you some advice in the words of Dr. Laura, "Go do the right thing."

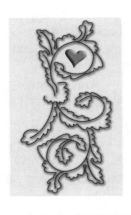

CHAPTER 12
Risky Business

I Just Can't Put My Finger On It

Don't misunderstand me. I am not against surgery always, but the surgical approach must never be a first option. We must recognize the limitations and shortcomings of modern heart treatments before rushing off to the hospital. The first thing to be wary of is misdiagnosis. Doctors still have a difficult time diagnosing heart disease because its symptoms vary so widely. The Framingham study, which observed more than 10,000 people over a thirty-year period, showed that one quarter of the heart attacks suffered were not recognized or treated.[1]

Another study showed that twenty-five percent of people who suffered a heart attack and went to the hospital were sent home. Additionally, forty percent of those admitted to the hospital for chest pains did not have heart disease.[2]

Just Because It Tastes Bad, Doesn't Mean It's Good For You

Many of us are under the erroneous assumption that a trip to the doctor's office is always a good thing. In regard to the treatment of heart disease, a doctor recently wrote in the *New England*

Journal of Medicine that, "there is growing evidence that more treatment is not always better and can actually be harmful."[3] It is widely recognized that invasive tests and treatments present significant risks. Yet, many doctors choose not to employ less invasive methods.

Mridu Gulati, M.D., said, "When it is difficult to establish a diagnosis, the first inclination is often to amass more data by performing increasingly sophisticated tests at the expense of a careful evaluation of the studies that have already been performed."[4] Doctors and patients should not view these tests and treatments as a cure-all.

For example, angiography is a method of putting a catheter into the heart through an artery in the groin or arm, injecting dye into the heart and then taking an x-ray of it so that the crown and arteries are visible. This method, while technologically pleasing and awe-inspiring, can hurt or even kill people. The catheter can clog the heart and provoke a heart attack, which is why a surgical team's presence is required whenever an angiography is performed.

When invasive and non-invasive treatments were compared to one another in a study, the results were astonishing. When 920 heart attack patients were tracked for nearly two years, with patients randomly divided into two groups and treated either surgically or non-invasively, the less invasively treated patients fared far better.[5]

Those who were treated with an invasive strategy had worse outcomes during the first year of follow-up. In addition, the number who died or who had another heart attack was significantly higher in the invasive-strategy group. Therefore, researchers determined that individuals suffering from a heart attack of the type studied do not benefit from routine, early invasive management.[6] Thomas Moore, a health policy analyst, writes, "Millions undergo hazardous treatment of undetermined benefit" and doctors continue to ignore the evidence suggesting that the benefits of these treatments is "significantly limited." [7]

One such set of procedures is coronary angiography and revascularization. These procedures have become standard fare for those suffering from heart disease. A recent article stated that many doctors "continue to believe that all patients with acute coronary syndromes are best treated with prompt coronary angiography and revascularization, despite the absence of scientific support for such an approach."[8] If you are a conspiracy theorist, there is an explanation for this phenomenon. The high cost of these procedures has created an economic boom that encourages their use. "The United States has an abundance of facilities for prompt angiography and revascularization and monetary remuneration to the facilities and physicians. The combination of these factors encourages the use of angiography and revascularization."[9]

Another popular procedure is coronary bypass graft surgery. One of the problems with bypass surgery is that it seems to speed up the rate at which affected arteries close up in the days that follow an operation. It also stops the body from creating "natural bypass" arteries. It is a known fact that the surgery itself harms the artery that is bypassed. Howard H. Wayne, a renowned cardiologist, said that the heart muscle "may actually be worse off following such surgery." He concludes that "the common practice of rushing patients in for emergency or urgent surgery because of a severely narrowed coronary artery is completely unnecessary."[10]

Not only are some of the thousands of bypasses performed each year unnecessary, they can also damage the brain. A recent study says that five years after having bypass surgeries, forty percent of the people tested showed a twenty percent drop in mental capacity. In other words, four in ten people lost one fifth of their brainpower.[11] Rushing into a bypass surgery without exploring less invasive options is a truly unwise decision.

Another modern treatment is the coronary stent. The coronary stent was just introduced in the 1990s, yet stent implantations are currently used in 60 to 70 percent of all interventional procedures. This sudden popularity is shocking when we con-

81

sider that "no study has shown that stents favorably influence mortality."[12]

Even angiograms are of questionable value. A recent study declares that angiograms don't provide enough information to help prevent heart attacks.[13] We are seeking solutions from technology and surgical innovation. We are looking for a silver bullet, but none exists.

Again, don't misunderstand me. I am not against heart surgery. Surgery can save our lives in a pinch. However, surgery is not a *cure* for heart disease. More research should be aimed at preventing and curing heart disease, instead of "bypassing" it.

Our search for a panacea has not gone unnoticed by the pharmaceutical industry either. An astounding number of drugs have been developed to lower blood pressure. Such drugs can save lives. But no drug can affect the underlying causes of heart disease. They are temporary band-aid solutions at best.

There is ample question whether these drugs are truly preventative measures. A recent study showed that people with the same levels of blood pressure vary widely in their susceptibility to heart disease.[14] Apparently, there is no ideal blood pressure. This doesn't mean we shouldn't try to lower our blood pressure, but we should be hesitant to embrace a drug solution.

The clinical evidence supporting the widespread use of surgical treatment and drug therapy in the prevention of heart disease is sparing at best. Yet, the popularity of the two avenues continues to grow. We should not rush toward the surgeon or the pharmacist when we can derive the same benefits through change in our exercise habit and our diet.

82

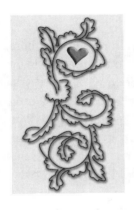

CHAPTER 13
Futuristic Therapies

The advances in heart care have been tremendous over the last 40 years but by no means is the quest for better solutions over. Researchers are just getting started and nothing is considered to be off limits. I will write about some of the newer technology that is now available to us in chapters 14 and 15 which include Ultrafast CT Scans, Ozone and natural therapies. In this chapter, I just want to touch on the seemingly outlandish that just may become mainstream one day in the future. Speaking of streams, let's talk about fish. Yes, fish, not the Omega 3's from fish oil; the actual fish. Zebra fish to be exact.

Zebra Fish
In December of 2002, a study was published in *Science* magazine about the research that is being done with Zebra fish.[1] What is the big deal about this little fish with black and white stripes? It has the ability to regenerate new cells to restore its heart completely after suffering any kind of damage to it. It can survive even if you were to cut out 20 percent of its heart.[2] Soon after the damage, its heart would repair itself to complete health.

There is extensive research on utilizing stem cells to produce healthy heart cells but Dr. Mark Keating of Harvard University believes that scientists should study different beings, like the Zebra fish, to discover what in their genetic codes allow them to regenerate heart cells.[3] Maybe a breakthrough like this would allow us to reprogram our genetic code to allow the heart to heal itself after a heart attack or something even more revolutionary. Maybe we could immunize the heart from attacks.

Other Animal Tricks

If you were told that you needed a heart transplant but there were no human hearts available. The only option that could be offered would be a monkey heart but the doctor's assured you that you could extend your life by twenty years guaranteed. Would you do it? In the future, this may be a decision that many will be faced with. Research started nearly twenty years ago in this area. In 1984, a team of medical scientists at Loma Linda University transplanted the heart of a baboon into a twelve-day-old baby girl, known as Baby Fae. The baby only lived twenty-one days after the procedure but the scientists proved that an animal heart could work, at least for a limited time, and they insist that the research should continue.[4] I am sure that your mind, as mine, is filled with ethical and moral questions about this.

Laser Show

Lasers are always exciting. Ronald Regan pumped millions of our tax dollars into his "Star Wars" defense program that promised to use lasers firing from satellites to destroy missiles, armed with nuclear warheads in the air before reaching their targets. Just recently, the military has reported successful use of land-based lasers to knock missiles down.

Lasers have been used successfully in the medical field as well. Who hasn't heard of laser eye surgery? I have already mentioned briefly how lasers are used during angioplasties but there is an even more intriguing use being tested.

A number of years ago, two cardiac surgeons visited me to show me their work using lasers. They said that they had developed an alternative to bypass surgery. Instead of using arteries from a different part of the body to go around damaged arteries and deliver blood to the heart muscle, they would simply use the laser to burn little passage ways right into the heart muscle. Imagine that your goal was to get water to a dry patch of land but the irrigation pipes were clogged. You could bypass the clog by using new pipe to go around the bad area and take water to the dry land or, you could just dig trenches into the land and let the water flow there naturally. The theory is fascinating. Keep a lookout in the news for future use of this technique.

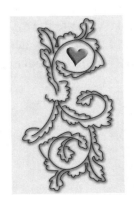

CHAPTER 14
State of the Heart Health Care

When I am out lecturing, I inevitably am approached by someone who has read one of my books and they ask me, "I have heard your advice and I agree with your approach but I am having a difficult time finding a doctor who will treat me the way that you describe. Do you actually treat patients or are you just an educator?" I always respond, there are many fine physicians in the world but if you are unable to locate one in your area, you may consider treatment options at my hospital the Oasis of Hope.

I believe that our heart program is the most comprehensive in the world. Why do I believe this? Simply because we offer the whole range of therapies from the conventional medical interventions including open heart surgery, angioplasty and advanced digital diagnostics to the alternative such as nutritional therapies, herbal remedies and Ozone therapies. We partner all of this with education, lifestyle counseling and even emotional and spiritual guidance.

I am sure that many renown cardiac surgeons and cardiologists who are accustomed to solving everything with knives and needles would not be so quick to congratulate us on our use of herbal remedies; and the naturopathic doctors who would like to juice every disease away are probably chilled that we actually

perform open heart surgery at our hospital; and the holistic heal-
ers who would like you to visualize yourself healthy don't really
see the value of digital scans. Let me explain why we are open to
so many methods. We acknowledge that the needs of patients
vary and that each type of medicine has its strengths and each has
its limitations. We focus on the patients needs and recommend
the best possible therapy for the specific condition of the patient.

My father who is now 87 years of age had a major heart
attack in 1985. He is closing in on 20 years that his life has been
extended. This would not have happened had it not been for
medical intervention. So much of his heart muscle was damaged
in his heart attack that the only solution was a pacemaker. Recently, he required a battery change and I hope they put in an
energizer bunny for it to keep going and going and going. His
doctors recommended a surgery to perform seven bypasses but
after we considered the fact that his heart was too damaged to
recover, we opted to avoid the surgery because it offered no benefit to him and the risk of death during surgery was very high.

In the case of my father-in-law, he had an angioplasty with
an installation of a stent to get the blood flowing to parts of his
heart that were damaged during his heart attack. He showed no
improvement and he had to undergo a series of tests, which finally
determined that the stent was functional, and the procedure was
successful but his heart was too damaged and scarred to respond.
He was determined to be inoperable and the doctors had nothing
left to offer him. We were quite concerned and not totally sure if
he would respond to alternative therapy but we brought him to
the Oasis of Hope and began our program. We started with
detoxification. Then we developed a exercise rehabilitation program with him and put him on our herbal supplement regimen. It
has now been two years and I am happy to say that he is alive and
well. Without alternative therapies, I am not sure that I could
have said the same thing. My wife is happy to still have her daddy!
My father would not have responded to alternative therapies. It

87

is conventional heart care that has kept him with us. For my father-in-law, no medical intervention could help him but the natural approach worked. This is why we make the whole range of treatment options available.

For the sake of organization, I will concentrate on medical procedures in this chapter. The next chapter will be dedicated to natural heart health boosters and the final chapter will concentrate on the emotional and spiritual issues that directly affect the health of heart.

Prevention

Heart disease is very preventable. In previous chapters I outline the things you can do to significantly lower your risk of a heart attack including diet, exercise and smoking cessation. In this chapter, I am sharing with you what we do with people who seek care at our hospital. In our local community, we are very involved in health education. We constantly lecture at parent/child conferences in schools as well as other forums. We also appear on television and radio interviews. When I say we, I mean a number of cardiologists who work at Oasis and myself. Our main message is that prevention is the only sure way to avoid an untimely death from a heart incidence. It is important for people to be proactive about preventing heart disease. We even go out to major companies and try to convince them to send their employees in for screening.

With everyone who comes in for a prevention or treatment program, we give to them the information contained in this book so that they can see the lifestyle changes that they need to make. I really believe that education has a far more powerful impact on health that medicine does. Then we go into diagnostics. All of our diagnostics are conventional.

Laboratory Examines

The blood tests that we do include a complete blood count and type of blood (i.e. A+), in order to evaluate the immune system and other illnesses. We do a blood chemistry work up of 24 parameters including renal and liver function, electrolytes and cholesterol index to evaluate the ratio between good and bad cholesterols. Another test is to determine the nutritional status of the patient.

Physical Examination/Clinical History
We conduct and interview with each patient as well as a physical examination for the expressed purpose of defining the needs of the patient. It is to determine the starting point and from there, we map out a treatment plan that will take the patient to a status of total health. As an important part of this exam, we determine the body mass index of each patient. In men, we also check prostate health and in women, we exam the breasts as well as take a pap smear.

Resting Electrocardiogram (EKG)
We conduct this test to establish the baseline of the anatomy of the patient's heart. In this process we are able to establish the size of the heart, condition of the ventricles and signs of previous myocardial heart attacks.

Stress Test
We put each patient on a treadmill with monitors that can detect myocardial ischemia (angina) in the coronary arteries. We also can detect electrical problems of the heart which would be arrhythmias (irregular heartbeats). The patient's overall physical condition under stress is also determined. We mainly measure the blood pressure and metabolic calories expended during the test.

X-Rays
One important point about the way medicine is approached at the Oasis of Hope is that even though a patient comes in for one problem, we do an overall evaluation of their health. Many times,

it can be a problem in an unsuspected place that is causing the illness in the heart. For this reason, we do a standard chest X-ray to evaluate the lungs and we do a sonogram of the abdomen to rule out any problems in the gallbladder, kidneys, pancreas, liver and intestinal tract.

Cardiac Scoring

One technology that I believe is one of the most powerful tools we have to determine the level of heart disease a person has and risk for a heart attack is the electron beam computerized tomography. You may have heard of these referred to as a fast CT scan. The machine that we have can take a scan of your heart and arteries in under one minute. It has a software program that enables it to take the images it compiles and generate a 3D image of your heart and arteries. Then, we can actually take a tour through your arteries on a video screen. We can see how blocked your arteries are getting. I recommend that everyone over the age of 40 have this scan done. I am now over 50 years of age and I recently had a scan done. I am happy to say that the results were not that bad. I am not at high risk but I was surprised to see that I do have signs of the beginning of arteriosclerosis. It is normal for my age but seeing it in three dimensional images was inspiring for me to keep up my exercise and Mediterranean diet.

A number of clinical trials conducted in institutions such as Mayo Clinic and UCLA indicate that the electron beam computerized tomography can help identify persons at high risk of a future heart incidence and that it is an effective diagnostic tool because it can detect calcifications in multiple vessels which correlate with obstructive disease such as arteriosclerosis. Our ultra fast CT scan is an effective non-invasive, non-exercise dependent test that is highly effective at detecting coronary artery disease.

Conventional Care

The Cardiovascular Institute at the Oasis of Hope is run by two of my colleagues who are cardiologists. They have a team that is

90

prepared to receive patients who are having mild discomfort, angina and cardiac arrest. They are experts at utilizing our digital catherization laboratory to intervene and do angiograms and angioplasty when necessary.

We also have a cardiac surgeon who was trained at the number one heart center in Mexico named the Ignacio Chavez Heart Institute. For major surgeries, we bring in another surgeon who is a professor at Ignacio Chavez because we are committed to providing the best care possible for our patients.

The only procedures that we are not currently utilizing are laser heart surgery, heart transplants and artificial hearts. We are currently studying the implementation of such procedures and I foresee that within the next ten years we will be able to provide these services as well.

Alternative Heart Therapies

I may not have delved into the conventional therapies the way my colleagues who are specialists in heart interventions would. This is merely because those types of surgical procedures are not my primary interest and since they are on board with us at Oasis, I will let them field questions in those areas. I do want to share with you quite a bit about alternative therapies for the heart however. They include herbal remedies and Ozone.

Ozone

There are so many new discoveries being made in the medical field today. It is hard to say what the future will be in heart care. What I can say with confidence however is that I won't be the least bit surprised if major breakthroughs will be in the use of oxygen, more specifically ozone which is an oxygen molecule made up of three oxygen atoms.

On a recent trip to Russia, I met with some scientists who took me to a hospital where they were infusing ozone into the veins of patients and they were getting excellent results lowering bad

91

cholesterol and decreasing plaque build up in the arteries. I have been using ozone for twenty years in the treatment of cancer but it never occurred to me to use it for heart health. I was amazed at the results and the science behind it. I am currently negotiating with the manufacturer of the ozone machine to export one from Russia to my hospital. I am hopeful that by the time this book is released in early 2003, we will already have the machine installed. The Russian scientists will be visiting our hospital to train our medical and nursing staff on the effective use of Ozone.

Ozone therapy has been used in many clinical situations for almost six decades since Wehrly and Steinbart described the procedure in 1954. Ozone has its pluses and its minuses when it comes to health. It can be therapeutic in the right amounts and damaging in the wrong amounts. In the stratosphere it acts as a shield from dangerous UV rays; but in the troposphere it is a major component of environmental photochemical smog that can harm humans, animals and plants.

As and oxidant, it can cause deleterious pulmonary and systemic effects when inhaled.[1] In contrast to its negative impact on the respiratory tract, human blood can tame ozone's strong oxidant properties allowing its therapeutic value to be utilized without acute nor chronic side effects. In layman's terms, we can't have a patient breathe ozone but we can safely introduce it into the blood.

Studies indicate that ozone therapy can be effective in treating chemotherapy-resistant infectious disease, chronic viral infections, immune deficiency syndromes, degenerative diseases of Central Nervous System (dementia senilis, Parkinson disease), orthopedic pathology and severe atheroclerotic lesions.[2] Other scientific reports indicate that under the right conditions, ozone therapy is safe and a powerful therapeutic agent.[3]

Here is where it gets really interesting. A study has found that ozone therapy can lower cholesterol levels and activate the antioxidant protections system in patients with myocardial infarction.

92

Results from other studies indicated that ozone therapy was safe and effective for patients with occlusive arteriorsclerosis of the lower limbs. Patients who participated in the study reported a reduction in total blood cholesterol and the ability to walk further without pain.[4] Another study was done with patients with occlusive arteriosclerosis of the lower limbs that could not undergo revascularizing surgery. They were given ozone therapy and experimented a significant decrease in both amputation percentage and the need pain controlling surgical procedures when compared to patients who did not receive ozone.[5]

I believe that ozone therapy could be used in conjunction with conventional therapies or as an alternative to patients who are inoperable. My research group will also be studying its value to prevent heart disease or prevent a recurrence of heart attack in patients who have already had one.

All of the treatments I have outlined in this chapter are done under the supervision of medical staff at the hospital. But what can you do at home as a part of your heart maintenance program? This is where we get into the area of supplements. In the next chapter, I outline the different herbs, vitamins and minerals that we use with all of our patients to help them prevent heart disease or to reverse their advanced cardiovascular conditions.

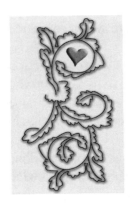

CHAPTER 15
Nature's Provision

The Heart of the Oasis of Hope Program

Another big part of our heart program is diet supplementation. Eating healthy is more than half of the ball game when you consider how to protect your heart naturally. But there are things that you probably wouldn't normally eat or eat in therapeutic quantities. There are substances in nature that can really help you prevent heart disease and we can use them in higher dosages to help people recover from a heart attack and lower their risk of a future incident. Let's go through some of the most heart friendly substances you can find.

NUTRIENTS

Coenzyme Q10

There are many medical publications that indicate the importance of Coenzyme Q10 (CoQ10). CoQ10 is vital to our body in the production of energy and heart health. As we age, our levels of CoQ10 begin to decline.[1] Smokers, people with heart disease and people with high levels of cholesterol also tend to be deficient in CoQ10.[2] CoQ10 can increase energy levels but more importantly, patients with chronic congestive heart failure and patients with acute myocardial infarction experience less complications and longer life expectancy.[3]

If you are over 40, for primary prevention I recommend that you take 50 mg daily of a typical commercially available form of coenzyme Q10 with your heaviest meal or take 30 milligrams a day of a new fully-solubilized form of coenzyme Q10 (Q-Gel) that possesses a high bioavailability (2.73 higher than the commercial forms).

For secondary prevention take 60 to 120 mg daily of Q-Gel (divided into two or three doses) or 200 mg per day of a commercial coenzyme Q10.[4]

L-Carnitine

L-carnitine, an amino acid, helps keep the heart beating properly. It also protects the heart muscle against oxygen deprivation and heart attack. [5]

L-carnitine can help you to avoid chest pains,[6] irregular heartbeat,[7] congestive heart failure,[8] high cholesterol[9] and peripheral vascular disease.[10]

You will also find that when you do any physical activity, you will have better stamina.[11] The extensive research of recent years indicates that L-carnitine can improve the exercise capacity of people who have suffered congestive heart failure, hypertensive heart disease or a heart attack.[12] L-carnitine also increases the ventricular contraction,[13] improves heart function and prolongs survival.[14] L-carnitine protects the myocardium against diphtheria toxin,[15] ischemia,[16] and myocardial infarction.[17] Lack of this amino acid keeps the heart from beating properly.[18]

For primary prevention, I suggest to take .5 to 1 gm of L-carnitine per day. For people who have already suffered a heart attack or have been diagnosed with congestive heart failure: 1 to 2 gm of L-carnitine should be used (divided into two or three doses).[19]

Taurine

Taurine, another very important amino acid helps the heart muscle to contract, and is useful in treating congestive heart failure.[20]

We give 2 or 3 grams of taurine a day to our patients who have been diagnosed with congestive heart failure or have had a heart attack. We usually give them 1 gram a couple times a day. The medical literature indicates that it is useful in the treatment of congestive heart failure.[21]

Taurine also lowers blood pressure[22] and strengthens heart muscle function.[23] Taurine has antioxidant effects[24] and has a role regulating myocardial contraction.[25]

HERBS

Hawthorn

Hawthorn fruit, flower and leaf extracts are known for the beneficial effects of increasing contractability of the heart muscle, improving cardiac efficiency, protecting against ischemia-induced ventricular arrhythmias, decreasing cholesterol blood levels, protecting against oxidative damage and reducing blood pressure. Hawthorn has also been shown to protect the heart from damage if it is ever deprived of oxygen.[26, 27]

In a clinical study it was shown that hawthorn extract increases exercise tolerance and quality of life in patients with congestive heart failure.[28]

I recommend 300 milligrams of hawthorn extract daily. For people who already have heart trouble, I recommend 600 to 900 milligrams per day divided into two to three doses.

Grape Seed Extract

Grape seed extract can really help to reduce the severity of a heart attack. It prevents cardiovascular disease by inhibiting platelet aggregation (reduces blood clots), capillary permeability and fragility and also by its antioxidant effects.[29]

The results from a recent study showed another important cardioprotective property of grape seed proanthocyanidin extract: its ability to block the death signal (apoptosis) of heart cells during ischemia.[30]

I recommend taking 100 to 150 milligrams of grape seed proanthocyanidin extract per day.

Ginkgo Biloba

The Ginkgo biloba tree is the oldest living being on earth. They are capable of living up to 4000 years. This wonderful tree is remarkably resistant to all kinds of pollution, plagues, virus and fungi and it can continue to reproduce up to an age of over 1,000 years.

Ginkgo biloba leaves contain active principles, especially flavonoids and a collection of unusual polycyclic structures which are unique in the vegetable kingdom called terpenoids (ginkgolides A and B). These terpenoids produce important cardioprotective effects, increasing the plasma antioxidant capacity[31] and increasing blood flow especially in deeper-seated medium and small arteries in the heart muscle,[32] inhibiting clot formation.[33] It also reduces the incidence of arrhythmias following ischemia.[34]

Ginkgo biloba is popular because it increases blood flow.[35] I recommend taking a daily dose of 120 milligrams of a Ginkgo biloba extract.

Garlic

Garlic lowers blood pressure, reduces cholesterol levels, reduces ventricular arrhytmias and prevents blood clotting. I recommend taking a daily dose equivalent to 4 grams of fresh garlic—the size of one large clove. Follow manufacturer's recommendations for commercial garlic and garlic-derived products. A good range is about 900 to 1200 milligrams per day of aged garlic extract.[36]

Garlic protects our heart in several ways. It lowers blood pressure, reduces cholesterol levels, reduces ventricular arrhythmias and prevents blood clotting. I recommend taking a daily dose equivalent to 4 grams of fresh garlic—the size of one large clove. Follow manufacture's interactions for commercial garlic and garlic-derived products. A good range is about 900 to 1200 milligrams per day of aged garlic extract.[37]

VITAMINS

The American Heart Association reports that taking multivitamins could prevent 50,000 heart disease deaths per year.[38] Doctors for the American Heart Association also stated, "Users of multi-vitamins have been reported to have reduced the prevalence of coronary artery disease compared with nonusers."[39] If you are like most people, then you are wondering, "Ok, but which vita-mins and minerals should I take?" A very recent study showed that dietary folic acid intake is an independent protective factor for myocardial infarction.[40]

B-Vitamins
The term Niacin refers to the two forms of vitamin B3, nicotinic acid and nicotinamide. High doses of vitamin B3 (1.2 to 2.0 grams per day) can reduce cholesterol levels by as much as 22 percent and lower triglycerides by 53 percent. Wait, there is more good news. This vitamin can also increase the good cholesterol by 33 percent and lower the rate of heart attack recurrence by nearly 30 percent. Scientific evidence suggests that vitamin B3 may reverse atherosclerosis to some extent.[41]

Vitamin B6 and folic acid have caught the attention of researchers. When taken in doses above the Recommended Daily Allowance, the studies found that B6 proved to be im-portant in the primary prevention of coronary heart disease by

98

lowering the level of homocysteine that is an amino acid which damages the inner layer of blood vessels.[42] Homocysteine is an enemy that can be fought with supplements. [43] This is very important when you consider that men with extremely high homocysteine levels are three times more likely to have an associated myocardial infarction.[44]

To me, the biggest case for B6 was the Nurses' Health Study that followed more than 80,000 women over 14 years.[45]

The results of the study were that women who have a high level of intake of vitamin B6 and folate lower their risk of CHD by 31 percent compared to women who have a low intake of vitamin B6 and folate. The lowest risk observed in the study was with intakes of folic acid above 400 mcg/day and vitamin B6 above 3 mg/day. This needs to get your attention because the average American consumes only 225 mcg/day.

Since B-vitamins work better together, I fully recommend a B-Complex supplement over consuming individual B-vitamins.

Vitamin C

Let's give a big cheer for vitamin C because it will do more to protect your heart that you will ever know. Vitamin C helps prevent the oxidation of bad cholesterol which helps in turn prevent atherogenesis. Another important benefit for coronary patients is that vitamin C helps the blood platelets to avoid sticking together.[46]

Recently, it was shown that vitamin C enhances the cardioprotective effects of the antioxidant glutathione.[47]

Here is the most powerful argument for vitamin C. "Individuals with the highest levels of vitamin C in their blood had only about half the risk of death ... than those with the lowest levels," said doctors from the University of Cambridge in a recent study.[48]

Here is where the saying "An apple a day keeps the doctor away" comes from – one apple (or orange) has enough vitamin C in it to help keep your heart healthy.[49]

Other studies point to further benefits if you can increase the blood content of vitamin C more so I recommend supplementing your diet with 2 or 3 grams a day.

Vitamin E

Here's the scoop on vitamin E. When it is taken in high doses, the risk of heart disease can decrease by as much as 43 percent. If you are taking medication to lower your cholesterol, catch this, people who take vitamin E in addition to their cholesterol-lowering drugs show less progression of heart disease than people who take only the drugs.[50]

In all of these vitamins, dosages are important to achieve the therapeutic effects. A study done over two years with close to 40,000 men who were taking a daily dose higher than 100 IU experienced a reduced risk of heart disease by 33 percent to 43 percent. Apparently, vitamin E slows down the hardening of our arteries by blocking the damaging effect of cholesterol.[51]

Vitamin E taken in high doses has been shown to reduce the risk of heart disease. Vitamin E is an antioxidant and has protective effects on the vasculature in people who have experienced heart failure.[52]

I recommend taking a daily supplement of 400 IU to 800 IU of vitamin E to help slow down if not stop the hardening of arteries.

MINERALS

Calcium

Low calcium intake is linked to high blood pressure. It may be that low serum calcium would increase the constriction of arterioles (reducing their diameter), which in turn increases arterial resistance to blood flow. As a result blood pressure is increased. A diet moderate to high in calcium content helps reduce and prevent high blood pressure.[53] Low-fat dairy products, fruit and vegetables can be great sources of calcium. Calcium, of course, is found in great quantities in dairy products but you need to watch the fat intake as well. Small amounts of low-fat milk, cheese and yogurt can be beneficial but consider other sources of calcium as well such as spinach.

One study showed that people who eat a lot of low-fat dairy products, fruit and vegetables and thus moderate to high content (aprox. 1200 mg/day) significantly reduce their blood pressure and prevent hypertension. [54]

Chromium

Because the oral dose of inorganic trivalent chromium has a low absorption rate, less than 2 percent, organically bonded chromium compounds which are more cell permeable have been developed.[55] The most intriguing of these is chromium picolinate, one of the best-absorbed sources of nutritional chromium, which is formed by a molecule of trivalent chromium bonded with three molecules of organic picolinic acid.[56] According to scientific studies, chromium picolinate is another wonderful bad cholesterol buster which makes it another substance I consider to be important for cardiovascular health.[57] Animal studies, as well as epidemiological correlations, provide additional evidence that good chromium nutrition may be antiatherogenic.[58] I suggest taking 200 to 400 mcg of chromium picolinate daily as a supplement.

Magnesium

Many times I have heard people say manganese when they really mean magnesium but if you are concerned about heart health, you definitely want to take magnesium. Not only is it necessary for everything the human body does, it may be particularly beneficial for people who have heart concerns or who have had a heart attack.[59]

The studies on heart health and magnesium dial right into its benefits in the areas of ischemic heart disease and cardiac arrhythmias.[60]

Analysis on the body of research on magnesium indicate that mortality may decrease following acute myocardial infarction for those consuming adequate quantities of magnesium. This has made it a fairly well accepted therapy for certain arrhythmias such as those provoked by ischemia and digitalis.[61] Whatever supplement you choose, make sure it contains magnesium.

At present, magnesium supplementation is well accepted as a therapy for certain arrhythmias such as those provoked by ischemia and digitalis or associated with heart failure.[62]

Potassium

You can ask any five-year-old what food is high in potassium and they will tell you bananas. Why does every one know that fact about bananas but we are hard put to say much else about any of the other food we eat? Well, that is another subject. Potassium helps the heart beat. A deficiency in potassium intake can help lead to high blood pressure. Taking potassium supplements usually can reduce your blood pressure.[63/64]

Everything that I have spoken of up to this point comes from nature's pharmacy. Why? Because they are effective and I really know of few drugs that I believe are beneficial. There is one made-made medication however that is remarkable. It is the crowned jewel of the pharmaceutical industry. You are going to be surprised. It's aspirin.

Aspirin

Of course you have used aspirin for headaches, muscle pain and fever but now we know that taking one tablet of aspirin every day decreases the number of heart attacks by as much as 40 percent.[65]

Aspirin helps blood platelets not stick together which helps avoid dangerous clots. Aspirin reduces the risk of a heart attack for people who suffer from angina.[66]

For people who have had a heart attack, they should take aspirin to help avoid an artery blocking clot.

In addition to thrombolytic agents, aspirin and heparin may also be administered. These drugs can prevent a clot in the artery from growing larger or from reforming after it has been dissolved by the thrombolytic agent. [67]

Aspirin is also effective at lowering the risk of stroke. It is important for men but it is also very helpful to help women avoid heart attacks according to a study conducted at Yale University. [68]

If your doctor does not want you to take aspirin because you are dealing with any type of gastrointestinal bleeding or ulcers, you can turn to omega -3 fatty acids. [69]

All of the vitamins, herbs and amino acids that I have presented here are readily available in health foods stores but I do want to give you a word of caution. Even though these are natural products, they can be as powerful as pharmaceuticals. You definitely want to consult a physician before you get yourself on a home program including these substances that we use as a part of the Oasis of Hope Heart Program. In the next chapter, we will move into the intangible aspects of heart health.

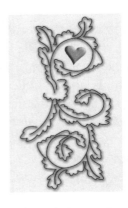

CHAPTER 16
Heart On Your Sleeve

Take a look at people around you. There are many people who really show their emotions and you can tell if they are generally content or if they are pretty much unhappy. Believe it or not, your emotional state has a dramatic effect on your heart health. It is written in an ancient book of wisdom and truth that a merry heart is good medicine and scientific studies agree with this. This is the reason that we try to build a relationship with our patients and find out what really makes their heart tick. Are they happy? Are they under a lot of stress? We try to find out what they are dealing with and then counsel them to help them find ways they can manage their emotions because if they don't, it could mean bad news for their heart. The main emotions that I want to talk about here are the negative ones fear, anger, worry and depression; and their powerful opponents love, faith and joy.

Fear, Anger and Worry
Fear, anger and worry are extremely stressful on your heart and in fact your whole body. These emotions trigger a chemical reaction in your body that is often referred to as "fight or flight." When you become suddenly afraid, angered or are worried, the sympathetic

nervous system (SNS) kicks in releasing hormones like adrenaline and norepinephrine. Hormones are tiny little things but they affect the body in powerful ways. If you doubt it, think about the last time you are some one close to you had PMS or suffered from menopause. When your body receives the burst of adrenaline and norepinephrine, it gets a quick boost of energy, strength and pain relief. This release of physical power, negation of pain, and mobilization of energy can actually save your life. In caveman times, it would help the Neanderthal slay the dinosaur or run away from it. This is what is happening when you hear of superhuman feats like one man lifting a car off of a child.

Stress is good on a temporary basis; the problem is that most people today are experiencing either fear, anger or worry all of the time. These stressful emotions cause arteries to constrict which makes the heart work harder. This is something I am sure you can relate to. What happens when you get angry, or when a police officer pulls you over, or when you are worried what your boss is going to say to you? Your heart starts pounding, right? Is this happening to you frequently? Heart disease used to be considered more common in people with type-A personalities—people who were competitive, perfectionist, impatient and prone to hostility. Now only type-H personalities—people who are overly-hostile—are believed to have higher risk for heart disease. A survey found that people who scored high on the hostility scale were seven times as likely to die by age fifty compared to their peers, and the difference was largely due to increased incidence of heart disease.[1]

Chronic activation of your SNS has the potential to harm you, for two reasons. One, it wears on your heart and circulation. Two, the systems in your body stop responding due to hyper-arousal. The first is wear and tear on your heart and circulation. The second happens when body systems shut down to fuel states of hyper-arousal.

A continual state of stress harms more than your heart, it can impact your digestion, immune-system activity, sexual drive, repair of tissues and gum health. It is linked to diabetes, chronic fatigue and cancer as well. The bottom line is that you need to get intense emotions under control.

Depression

A study published in July 1998 issue of *Archives of Internal Medicine* has linked depression to coronary disease. Another study published in *Circulation* in 1996 reported that people who had a two-week mild depression also had twice the risk of heart disease; a history of more serious depression quadrupled the risk. Another Circulation study showed up to a 70 percent higher risk for heart disease in depressed people. Depression affects the way your nervous system regulates your heart rate and blood vessel activity. Depressed people tend to have faster heart rates, higher blood pressure, and "stickier" platelets (clotting components) in their blood.

I hope all of this information is not starting to get you scared, angry, worried or depressed. On the contrary, I want you to know that there are wonderful ways to counteract these negative emotions.

STRESS BUSTERS

Love

If you have a loving relationship, you will have less heart problems than if you are in an unhappy relationship. Women who reported marital dissatisfaction were more likely than satisfied women to have significant plaque build-up in the main artery of the heart. They were also more likely to have blockages in the carotid arteries in the neck, a known risk factor for stroke.

Unhappiness in a marriage may harm the heart by inflicting "wear and tear" on the body, said one of the study's authors. Like stress in general, marital dissatisfaction may lead to habitual elevations in heart rate, blood pressure and stress hormones.[2]

How important is love? Dean Ornish in his book, *Love & Survival* (HarperCollins, 1998), wrote that, "I am not aware of any other factor in medicine—not diet, not smoking, not exercise, not stress, not genetics, not drugs, not surgery—that has a greater impact on our quality of life, incidence of illness and premature death from all causes."[3]

That morning kiss goodbye before going to work is more important than you ever imagined!

Faith

One of the most important ways you can decrease fear is to increase faith. Countless studies from Duke University indicate that people that have some sort of religious faith recover better from illness. One study conducted at Duke with heart patients indicated that those who were prayed for recovered better and had less complications than those who were not prayed for.

Let me explain a little about faith. Faith is a belief in a power higher than yourself. Fear and worry often result because of a lack of resources. If you have to pay $500.00 rent and you have only $300.00, your fear and worry increase. Right now with terrorism, we fear on an individual level that our federal agents, police and soldiers may not be able to protect us from attack. Here is where faith comes in. We tap into a being that has more resources than us. We believe in an Almighty that has unlimited resources and is completely able to resolve every problem. As a Christian, I walk with a sense of security because I believe that God is able to protect me, and, if something bad should happen, He will take me to a better place. If you personally don't believe in God, that is to say that you don't have faith, I suggest you find some faith because it has a positive effect on your physical health as well.

Joy

One of my favorite studies in the world indicates that one minute of anger depresses the immune system for six hours. On the other hand, one minute of laughter stimulates the immune system for 24 hours!

Mind over Matter

In this chapter we see that your emotions can either hurt or help you. Your mind truly affects physical matter. I do want to mention however that your body can also affect your mind in a positive way.

Recently a study was conducted that involved 156 people suffering from depression. The group was divided into three groups.

- One group was given antidepressants only.
- One group was given antidepressants plus group aerobics (thirty minutes, three times a week).
- One group was not given antidepressants but was put on an exercise regimen.

After nine months, only thirty percent of those in the exercise-only group were still depressed while more than half of the people in the other groups were depressed.

Doing only fifty minutes of exercise a week has been shown to cut your chances of being depressed in half, and many studies show cognitive behavioral therapy can be as effective as drugs.[4]

Don't Get Too Excited

Good news and bad news can translate into stress on your heart. I remember a joke about a woman whose husband had heart troubles. The man would send her every day to by a lottery ticket but one day, they had the winning number and the payout was $30 million dollars! She was afraid that the news would shock her husband into a heart attack so she called her pastor. She knew that he could break the good news to her husband gently. The pastor went into see the man and asked, "Let's suppose that you won $30 million in the lottery. What would you do with the money?" The man responded, "I would donate it all to your church pastor." The pastor died right there of a heart attack!

Sports

Sometimes the suspense of a sports game gets intense in the last moments, especially if the teams are tied. It is common to call those games "cardiac games." I have news for you. It is more than an expression. A recent study measured the incidence of heart attacks after soccer games that went into the penalty phase. This occurs when the teams are tied at the end of regulation time and they have to decide the game with a shoot out of penalty shots. The scientists were from the University of Bristol and the University of Birmingham and the game that was studied was when England played against Argentina in the World Cup in 1998. It was reported in the *British Medical Journal* that the incidence of heart attack increased by 25 percent in England the following day after the English team sustained an emotional loss to the Argentines in the penalty phase. I don't know what to tell you except take it easy, it's just a game. But for many sports fans, it is a life or death issue if their team wins or loses, literally. [5]

REFERENCES

Chapter 1
Know Your Enemy

[1] The Franklin Institute Science Museum, www.fi.edu

[2] "Leading causes of death 1900–1978," National Center for Health Statistics. Hyattsville, Maryland: Public Health Service.

[3] See note 1.

[4] See note 2.

[5] Thomas Jefferson University Hospital.jeffersonhospital.org/hearts/show.asp?durki=4017

[6] American Heart Association, www.americanheart.org

[7] See note 5.

[8] See note 1.

[9] Michael H. Crawford, M.D., Robert S. Flinn Prof. and Chief, Division of Cardiology, Univ. of New Mexico School of Medicine, «Heart,» *World Book Encyclopedia,* 1998, Chicago, Ill., software version 1.0

[10] Ibid.

[11] Ronald M. Lauer, et al., «National Cholesterol Education Program,» Pediatrics, Burlington, Vermont. March 1992, p. 530.

[12] Charles A. Andersen, M.D., (Chief of Vascular Surgery Service, Tripler Army Medical Center), «Understanding your atherosclerosis and living with it,» *Iowa Health Book: Internal Medicine*

110

[13] Barry L. Zaret, *Yale University School of Medicine Heart Book* (New York: William Morrow and Company, Inc.), p. 136.

[14] Ibid.

[15] Ibid, p. 143.

[16] Ibid.

[17] Ibid.

Chapter 2
Friend Or Foe?

[1] Reuters Ltd. 1998, http://www.heartinfo.org/reuters2000/t021622f.htm

[2] Michael R. Eades and Mary Dan Eades, *Protein Power* (New York: Bantam), p. 362.

[3] Ibid, 392.

[4] Ibid, 362–364.

[5] Uffe Ravnskov, M.D., "The Cholesterol Myths," home.swipnet.se/~w-25775/

[6] "Locating Gene that Explains Cholesterol Absorption," University of Texas Southwestern Medical Center, 9/1/98, www.newswise.com/articles/1998/9/ABSORB.SWM.html

[7] Thomas J. Moore, *Heart Failure: A Critical Inquiry into American Medicine and the Revolution in Health* Care (New York: Random House), p. 72

[8] See note 5.

[9] See note 5

[10] Barry Sears, Ph.D., *The Zone*, (New York: HarperCollins), p. 142

Chapter 3
Up In Smoke

[1] Ira S. Ockene et al. «A statement for healthcare professionals from the American Heart Association,» April 1997, www.americanheart.org

[2] «Cigarette smoking-attributable mortality and years of potential life lost — United States, 1990,» August 27, 1993 /

42(33);645–649. http://www.cdc.gov/epo/mmwr/preview/mmwrhtml/00021441.htm

[3] Denise Pinney, «Understanding the connection between smoking and heart disease. Smoking eries, Part 1,» Reuters Ltd., Center for Cardiovascular Education, Inc. www.heartinfo.org

[4] American Heart Association «Cigarette smoking, cardiovascular disease, and stroke: A statement for healthcare professionals from the American Heart Association,» *Circulation.*—1997; 96:3243–3247.

[5] «Smoking said to promote blood clots.» Reuters Ltd., Center for Cardiovascular Education, Inc. www.heartinfo.org

[6] 12WKRC, Cincinnati, Ohio. www.thehealthauthority.com/commons/heartcare/help_your_heart04.cfm

[7] «Every cigarette takes 11 minutes off man's life,» Source: *British Medical Journal* 2000;320:53. Reuters Ltd., Center for Cardiovascular Education, Inc. www.heartinfo.org

[8] «Cigar smoking: An unsafe alternative to cigarettes,» Sources: «Cigars to not have the same restrictions as cigarettes,» *American Cancer Society News Today*—June 2000. Reuters Ltd., Center for Cardiovascular Education, Inc. www.heartinfo.org

[9] Ibid.

[10] Thomas Jefferson University Hospital, www.jeffersonhospital.org/hearts/show.asp?durki=4017

[11] http://www.smokeaway.org/whyquit.htm Tobacco or Health: A Global Status Report, Geneva, Switzerland: World Health Organization [WHO], 1997) cited at_http://www.americanheart.org/statistics/riskfactors.html#smoke

Chapter 4
Learning To Say "No"

[1] Rex Russell, *What the Bible Says About Healthy Living,*, Ventura, California: Regal Books, p. 177.

[2] Ibid.

[3] Alberto Ascherio, M.D., et al., «Trans Fatty Acids and

Coronary Heart Disease,» *New England Journal of Medicine*, June 24, 1999, p. 1997

4 Ely DL, "Overview of dietary sodium effects on and interactions with cardiovascular and neuroendocrine functions", *American Journal of Clinical Nutrition* 65, Supplement (1997):594S-605S.

5 Ibid.

6 Chrysant GS et al. "Dietary salt reduction in hypertension – what is the evidence and why is it still controversial?", *Progress in Cardiovascular Diseases* 42, no.1 (1999):23-38.

7 JG Fodor et al., "Recommendations on dietary salt", *Canadian Medical Association Journal* 160, Supplement 9 (1999):S29-S34.

8 See notes 6 and 7.

9 www.meatstinks.com, PETA

Chapter 5
Take A Load Off

1 "Obesity continues climb in 1999 among american adults," March 23, 2001, http://www.cdc.gov/nccdphp/dnpa/probesity.htm

2 Suzanne Rostler, «Americans in denial about weight and risks of obesity,» Reuters Ltd., Center for Cardiovascular Education, Inc. www.heartinfo.org

3 U.S. Department of Health and Human Services, *The Surgeon General's Report on Nutrition and Health* (New York: Warner Books), p. 11.

4 Erin Bried, *Self* (New York) 12/2000, pp. 160–161

5 Jerome Kassirer, "Losing weight—an Ill-fated New Year's resolution," *New England Journal of Medicine*, (Boston, Mass.: Massachusetts Medical Society), January 1, 1998, p. 53

6 JE Manson et al. "Body weight and mortality among women," *New England Journal of Medicine*. 1995; 333:677–685.

7 Thomas Jefferson University hospital, www.jeffersonhospital.org/hearts/show.asp?durki=4017

[8] Adapted from Obesity Education Initiative: National Institutes of Health, National Heart, Lung, and Blood Institute, "Clinical guidelines on the identification, evaluation, and treatment of overweight and obesity in adults,", Preprint June 1998, www.americanheart.org

[9] L Lapidus et al. "Distribution of adipose tissue and risk of cardiovascular disease and death: a 12 year follow up of participants in the population study of women in Gothenburg, Sweden," *British Medical Journal.* 1984;289:1257–1261. B Larsson et al. "Abdominal adipose tissue distribution, obesity, and risk of cardiovascular disease and death: 13 year follow up of participants in the study of men born in 1913," *British Medical Journal,* 1984;288:1401–1404.

[10] Lynn Grieger, «Body Fat Distribution and Heart Disease Risk in Children and Adolescents,» http://www.heartinfo.org/news99/fatdist030399.htm

[11] "Cholesterol and children," WellnessWeb, www.wellweb.com/smart/aahtchil.htm

[12] «National Cholesterol Education Program,» *Pediatrics*, March 1992, p. 530.

[13] The Bogalusa Heart Study, p. 2

[14] Richard P. Troiano, PhD et al. «Overweight prevalence and trends,» *Arch. Pediatr. Adolesc. Med.*, October 1995, pg. 1085, 1088.

[15] See note 10.

[16] «Exercise, lipids, and obesity in adolescents of parents with premature coronary disease,» http://www.jhbmc.jhu.edu/cardiology/partnership/kids/chdchildren/tsld034.htm

[17] Gerald S. Berenson, M.D, et al. «Association between multiple cardiovascular risk factors and atherosclerosis in children and young adults,» *New England Journal of Medicine*, June 4, 1998, p. 1655

[18] Ibid.

[19] «Cholesterol-lowering diets and effects on children,» *Nutrition Today,* March 2000, www.findarticles.com/m0841/2_35/62083816/p1/article.jhtml

Chapter 6
Other Culprits

[1] Artemis P. Simopoulos, M.D. and Jo Robinson, *The Omega Plan* (New York: HarperCollins), 1998, p. 51.
[2] Barry L. Zaret et al. Yale University School of Medicine Heart book, (New York: William Morrow and Company, Inc.),157.
[3] Ibid.
[4] The Franklin Institute Science Museum, www.fi.edu
[5] Alicia Marie Belchak, "Exercise reduces heart disease risk among diabetics," Sources: *Annals of Internal Medicine* 2001;134:96–106. Reuters Ltd., Center for Cardiovascular Education, Inc. www.heartinfo.org
[6] «Heart disease rates drop for all but diabetics.» Sources: The *Journal of the American Medical Association* 1999;281:1291–1297. Reuters Ltd., Center for Cardiovascular Education, Inc. www.heartinfo.org
[7] Emma Patten-Hitt, «Diabetic arteries often re-close after surgery.» Sources: *Circulation* 2001;103:1218–1224, 1185–1187. Reuters Ltd., Center for Cardiovascular Education, Inc. www.heartinfo.org
[8] Harvey Black, «The connection between oral health and other health,» WebMD, p. 2, onhealth.webmd.com/conditions/in-depth/item/item%2C37240_1_1.asp
[9] Ibid.
[10] Judy Siegel-Itzkovich, «Gum disease can ruin far more than your smile,» *Jerusalem Post*, June 25, 2000, p. 4, www.jpost.com/Editions/2000/05/21/Health/Health.6989.html
[11] Randolph Fillmore, «Gum disease may be a threat to the heart,» WebMD, p. 2, onhealth.webmd.com/conditions/in-depth/item/item «Another reason to see the dentist,» WebMD, 9/27/99, p. 1 onhealth.webmd.com/conditions/briefs/item%2C50352.asp
[12] Ibid.
[13] Eurekalert, «Low dietary vitamin C can increase the risk

for periodontal disease, especially in smokers,»
www.eurekalert.org/releases/aap-ldv081400.html

Chapter 7
Back To Basics

[1] Julie Brussell, «Traditional Foods, Unconventional Wisdom,» *Conscious Choice*, September 2000, www.consciouschoice.com/issues/cc1309/traditionalfoods1309.html

[2] Sally Fallon, «Nasty, brutish and short,» *The Weston A. Price Foundation*, www.westonaprice.org/nasty_brutish_short.htm

[3] Staffan Lindeberg, «On the Benefits of Ancient Diets,» www.panix.com/~paleodiet/lindeberg/

[4] Riccardo Baschetti, «Diabetes in aboriginal populations,» *Canadian Medical Association Journal* 2000;162:969, Padua, Italy, www.cma.ca/cmaj/vol-162/issue-7/0969a.htm

[5] Press Release, «Traditional Chinese Diet Helps Ward Off Heart Disease,» www.cuhk.edu.hk/ipro/991110e.htm

[6] Sarah Yang, «Mediterranean diet still healthy when authentic, not Americanized,» CNN.com republished article by WebMD, www2.cnn.com/2000/FOOD/news/05/01/mediterranean.eating.wmd/index.html

[7] A Trichopoulou, and P Lagiou, "Healthy traditional Mediterranean diet: An expression of culture, history and lifestyle", Nutrition Reviews 55, no.11 (1997):383-389.

[8] Ibid.

Chapter 8
A Healthy Appetite

[1] U.S. Department of Health and Human Services, The Surgeon General's Report on Nutrition and Health, Warner Books, New York, p. 2

[2] Ibid.

[3] Ibid. p. 6.

[4] Ibid. p. 19

Chapter 9
Eat To The Beat Of A Different Drum

[1] S Bengmark, "Ecoimmunonutrition: a challenge for the third millennium", *Nutrition* 14, no.7–8 (1998):563–572.

[2] MW Gillman, et al., "Protective effect of fruits and vegetables on development of stroke in men", *Journal of the American Medical Association* 273, (1995):1113–1117.

[3] *New England Journal of Medicine* 1/6/2000, p. 7

[4] Dean Ornish, M.D., "Low-Fat Diets," *New England Journal of Medicine,* DATE UNKNOWN, vol. 338, no. 2, p. 127

[5] CL Vecchia et al. "Vegetable consumption and risk of chronic disease", *Epidemiology* 9, (1998):208–210.

[6] F Sacks, et al., "A dietary approach to prevent hypertension: A review of the dietary approaches to stop hypertension (DASH) study", *Clinical Cardiology* 22, Supplement III (1999):III-6–III-10.

[7] BV Howard and D Kritchevsky, "Phytochemicals and cardiovascular disease: a statement for health care professionals from the American Heart Association", *Circulation* 95, (1997):2591–2593.

[8] CV De Whalley et al. "Flavonoids inhibit the oxidative modification of low-density lipoproteins by macrophages", *Biochemistry and Pharmacology* 39, (1990):1743-1750. J. Robak and RJ Gryglewski, "Flavonoids are scavengers of superoxide anion", *Biochemistry and Pharmacology* 37, (1988):83–88.

[9] MGL Hertog et al. "Dietary antioxidant flavonoids and risk of coronary heart disease: the Zutphen elderly Study", *The Lancet* 342, (1993):1007–1011.

[10] RA Nagourney, "Garlic: Medicinal food or nutritious medicine?", *Journal of Medicinal Food* 1, no. 1 (1998):13-28.

[11] WJ Graig , "Phytochemicals: Guardians of our health", *Journal of the American Dietetic Association* 97, Supplement 2 (1997):S199-S204.

[12] PN Appleby et al. "The Oxford Vegetarian Study: an over-

117

view", *American Journal of Clinical Nutrition* 70, Supplement (1999):525S–531S.

[13] EJ Schaefer and ME Brosseau, "Diet, lipoproteins, and coronary heart disease", *Endocrinology and Metabolism Clinics of North America* 27, no.3 (1998):711–732.

[14] EJ Schaefer, and ME Brosseau, "Diet, lipoproteins, and coronary heart disease", *Endocrinology and Metabolism Clinics of North America* 27, no.3 (1998):711–732.

[15] GM Wardlaw and TJ Snook , "Effect of diets high in butter, corn oil, or high-oleic acid sunflower oil or serum lipids and apolipoproteins in men", *American Journal of Clinical Nutrition* 51, (1990):815–822.

P Mata et al. "Effect of dietary monounsaturated fatty acids on plasma lipoproteins and apolipoproteins in women", *American Journal of Clinical Nutrition* 56, (1992):77–83.

Chapter 10

A Real Meal Deal

[1] F Visioli et al. "Low density lipoprotein oxidation is inhibited in vitro by olive oil constituents", *Atherosclerosis* 117, (1995):25–32.

F Visioli et al. "Free radial-scavenging properties of olive oil polyphenols", *Biochem. Biophys. Res. Comm.* 247, (1998):60–64.

[2] "Olive oil may reduce need for blood pressure drugs." Sources: *Archives of Internal Medicine* 2000;160:837–842. Reuters Ltd., Center for Cardiovascular Education, Inc. www.heartinfo.org

[3] GE Fraser, "A possible protective effect of nut consumption on risk of coronary heart disease", Archives of *Internal Medicine* 152,(1992):1416–1424.

L Brown et al. "Nut consumption and risk of recurrent coronary heart disease (abstract)", *The FASEB Journal* 13, no. (4–5) (1999):A538.

[4] GE Fraser et al. "Effect of risk factor values on lifetime risk of an age at first coronary event", *American Journal of Epidemiology* 142, (1995):746–758.

[5] D Steinberg and A Lewis, "Oxidative modification of

LDL and atherogenesis", *Circulation* 95, (1997):1062–1071.

[6] JG Keevil et al., "Grape juice, but not orange juice or grapefruit juice, inhibit human platelet aggregation", *Journal of Nutrition* 130, (2000):53–56.

[7] R Sauter et al. "Purple grape juice inhibits platelet function and increases platelet-derived nitric oxide release", *Circulation* 98, (1998):581–585.

[8] WB Kannel and RC Ellison, "Alcohol and coronary heart disease: The evidence for a protective effect", Clin. Chim. Acta 246, (1996):59–76.

[9] DR Lowry et al. "Alcohol consumption and incidence of hypertension. The John Hopkins Precursors Study", *Circulation* 92, no.8 (1995):619.

[10] GJ Soleas et al. "Wine as a biological fluid: History, production, and role in disease prevention", *Journal of Clinical Laboratory Analysis* 11, (1997):287–313.

[11] SV Nigdikar et al. "Consumption of red wine polyphenols reduces the susceptibility of low–density lipoproteins to oxidation in vivo", *American Journal of Clinical Nutrition* 68, (1998):258-265.

[12] S Renaud and de M Lorgeril, "Wine, alcohol, platelets and the French paradox for coronary heart disease", *The Lancet* 339, (1992):1523-1526.

[13] JM Geleijnse et al. "Tea flavonoids may protect against atherosclerosis: The Rotterdam Study", *Arch. Inter. Med. 159,* (1999):2170-2174.

[14] AA Hakim et al. "Coffee consumption in hypertensive men in older middle-age and the risk of stroke: The Honolulu Heart Program", *Journal of Clinical Epidemiology* 51, no.6 (1998):487-494.

[15] M Woodward and H Tunstall-Pedoe, "Coffee and tea consumption in the Scottish Heart Health Study follow-up: conflicting relations with coronary risk factors, coronary disease, and all cause mortality", *Journal of Epidemiology Community Health* 53, (1999):481–487.

[16] C Sanbongi et al. "Polyphenols in chocolate, which have

antioxidant activity, modulate immune functions in humans in vitro", *Cellular Immunology* 177, (1997):129–136.

[17] AL Waterhouse, et al., "Antioxidants in chocolate", *The Lancet* 348, (1996):834.

[18] EB Rimm, et al., "Vegetable, fruit, and cereal intake and risk of coronary heart disease among men", *Journal of the American Medical Association* 275, (1996):447–451.

[19] GE Fraser, et al., "A possible protective effect of nut consumption on risk of coronary heart disease. The Adventist Health Study", *Archives in Internal Medicine* 152, (1992):1416–1424.

[20] KA Meyer et al. "Whole-grain intake may reduce the risk of ischemic heart disease death in postmenopausal women: the Iowa Women's Health Study", *American Journal of Clinical Nutrition* 68, (1998):248–257.

[21] S Liu et al. "Whole-grain consumption and risk of coronary heart disease: results from the Nurses' Health Study", *American Journal of Clinical Nutrition* 70, (1999):412–419.

[22] L Sampson et al. "Methodological considerations in applying metabolic data to an epidemiologic study using a semi-quantitative food frequency questionnaire", *European Journal of Clinical Nutrition* 52, (1998):S87.

[23] WE Connor, "Importance of n-3 fatty acids in health and disease", *American Journal o Clinical Nutrition* 71, Supplement (2000):171S–175S.

[24] MK Copass "Dietary intake of long-chain n-3 polyunsaturated fatty acids and the risk of primary cardiac arrest", *American Journal of Clinical Nutrition* 71, Supplement (2000):208S–212S.

Bang HO et al. "The composition of the Eskimo food in north western Greenland", *American Journal of Clinical Nutrition* 33, (1980):2657–2661.

[25] MK Copass et al. "Dietary intake of long-chain n-3 polyunsaturated fatty acids and the risk of primary cardiac arrest", *American Journal of Clinical Nutrition* 71, Supplement (2000):208S–212S.

[26] H Shimokawa and PM Vanhoutte, "Dietary omega-3 fatty

acids and endothelium-dependent relaxations in porcine coronary arteries", *American Journal of Physiology* 256, (1989):H968–H973.

[27] P Artemis et al. *The Omega Plan* (New York: HarperCollins) 1998, p. 52–53, 102.

[28] FN Hepburn et al. "Provisional tables on the content of omega-3 fatty acids and other fat components of selected foods", *Journal of the American Diet Association* 86, (1986):788–793.

SL Connor and WE Connor. "Are fish oils beneficial in the prevention and treatment of coronary artery disease?", *American Journal of Clinical Nutrition* 66, Supplement (1997):1020S–1031S.

[29] JX Kang and A Leaf, "Prevention of fatal arrhythmias by polyunsaturated fatty acids", *American Journal of Clinical Nutrition* 71, Supplement (2000):202S–207S.

[30] DS Siscovick et al. "Dietary intake and cell membrane levels of long-chain n-3 polyunsaturated fatty acids and the risk of primary cardiac arrest", *Journal of the American Medical Association* 274, (1995):1363–1367.

[31] ML Burr et al, "Effects of changes in fat, fish, and fiber intakes on death and myocardial reinfarction: Diet and Reinfarction Trial (DART)". *The Lancet* 2, (1989):756–761

[32] M De Lorgeril et al. "Mediterranean alpha-linolenic acid-rich diet secondary prevention of coronary heart disease", *The Lancet* 343, (1994):1454–1459.

[33] VA Ajani et al. "Fish consumption and risk of sudden cardiac death", *Journal of the American Medical Association* 279, (1998):23–27.

[34] WE Connor , "Importance of n-3 fatty acids in health and disease", *American Journal o Clinical Nutrition 71*, Supplement (2000):171S–175S. DS Siscovick, et al., "Dietary intake of long-chain n-3 polyunsaturated fatty acids and the risk of primary cardiac arrest", *American Journal of Clinical Nutrition 71*, Supplement (2000):208S–212S.

121

35   PM Kris-Etherton, et al., "Polyunsaturated fatty acids in the food chain in the United States", *American Journal of Clinical Nutrition 71*, supplement (2000):179S–188S.

36   Artemis P. Simopoulos, M.D., and Jo Robinson, *The Omega Plan* (New York: HarperCollins) 1998, p. 52

Chapter 11
Get A Move On

1   AP, «Study: Healthy living slashes heart risks,» *Dallas Morning News,* Nov. 9, 1999, 3A.

2   Ibid.

3   A. La Voie, "Vigorous exercise lowers risk factors more than moderate activity," *Medical Tribune* (Family Physician Edition) 1997; February 20:38;(4):5; www.thrive.net/health/Library/CAD/abstract1284.

4   J. E. Brody, "Study says exercise must be strenous to add to lifespan," *New York Times*, April 19, 1995, 144; (50,036):A1, B7, www.thrive.net/health/Library/CAD/abstract4429.

5   Janice C. Wright, "Gains in life expectancy from medical interventions—Standardizing data on outcomes," *New England Journal of Medicine,* August 6, 1998, pp. 380–385.

6   "Women put best foot forward to reduce heart disease, stroke risk," American Heart Association, www.americanheart.org/whats_News_AHA_News_Releases/manson.htm

Chapter 12
Risky Business
I Just Can't Put My Finger On It

1   Thomas Moore, *Heart Failure* (New York: Random House), p. 153.

Louise Williams, «Framingham Heart Study Celebrates 50 Years,»NIH Record 11/17/98, www.nih.gov/news/NIH-Record/11_17_98/story06.htm

2   L. Kristin Newby, M.D. et al., "The Chest-Pain Unit—Ready for Prime Time?"; *New England Journal of Medi-*

cine; December 24, 1998, p. 1930

[3] Lisa M. Schwartz, et al. "Misunderstanding about the effects of race and sex on physicians' referrals for cardiac catheterization," *New England Journal of Medicine*, July 22, 1999, p. 281.

[4] Mridu Gulati, M.D., et al. "Impatient Inpatient Care;" *New England Journal of Medicine*; January 6, 2000: 39, 40.

[5] «America's #1 Killer,» pp. 4, references *New England Journal of Medicine*, June 18, 1998.

[6] William E. Boden, «Outcomes in patients with acute non-Q-wave myocardial infarction randomly assigned to an invasive as compared with a conservative management strategy,» *New England Journal of Medicine*, Massachusetts Medical Society, Boston, Mass. June 18, 1998, http://www.nejm.org/content/1998/0338/0025/1785.asp

[7] Thomas Moore, *Heart Failure*, (Random House: New York), pp. 270–271.

[8] *New England Journal of Medicine*, June 18, 1998, «Use and overuse of angiography and revascularization for acute coronary syndromes.» http://www.nejm.org/content/1998/0338/0025/1838.asp

[9] Ibid

[10] Howard H. Wayne, M.D., F.A.C.C., F.A.C.P «Living longer with heart disease: The noninvasive approach that will save your life,». http://www.heartprotect.com/mortality-stats.shtml

[11] «Loss of brainpower after bypass may last,» *USA Today*, 2/8/2001, 10D; na.

[12] Alice K. Jacobs, M.D., "Coronary stents—Have they fulfilled their promise?" *New England Journal of Medicine*, December 23, 1999, Massachusetts Medical Society, Boston, Mass. http://www.nejm.org/content/1999/0341/0026/2005.asp

[13] Howard H. Wayne, M.D., F.A.C.C., F.A.C.P "Angiograms,". http://www.heartprotect.com/angiograms.shtml

[14] Peggy C.W. Van Den Hoogen et al., «The relation between blood pressure and mortality due to coronary heart disease

among men in different parts of the world,» *The New England Journal of Medicine,* 1/6/2000 Massachusetts Medical Society, Boston, Mass., p. 7.

Chapter 13
Futuristic Therapies

[1] "How Zebrafish mend damaged hearts" *Science.* Vol. 298, No. 5601. December 2002. www.sciencemag.org

[2] "Zebrafish may hold the key to heart repair" http://www.cnn.com/2002/HEALTH/12/12/self.mending.heart.ap/index.html

[3] Ibid.

[4] The Franklin Institute Science Museum, www.fi.edu

Chapter 14
State of the Heart Health Care

[1] WA Pryor et al., "The cascade mechanisms to explain ozone toxicity: The role of lipid ozonation products," *Free Rad. Biol. Med.* 1995,19:935-941.

[2] V Bocci, "Biological and clinical effects of ozone. Has ozone therapy a future in medicine?", *Br. J. Biomed. Sci.* 1999;56:270-280.

[3] N Di Paolo et al., "Extracorporeal blood oxygenation and ozonation (EBOO) in man. Preliminary report." *International J. Artificial Organs* 2000,23(2):131-141. Hernández F et al. "Decrease of blood cholesterol and stimulation of antioxidative response in cardiophathy patients treated with endovenous ozone therapy." *Free Rad. Biol. Med.* 1995,19(1):115-119.

[4] T Tylicki et al., "Beneficial clinical effects of ozonated autohemotherapy in chronically dialysed patients with atherosclerotic ischemia of the lower limbs-pilot study," *Int. J. Artif, Org.* 2001, 24(2):79-82. B Turczynski et al., "Ozone therapy and viscosisty of blood and plama, distance of intermittent claudication and certain biochemical plasma components in patients with occlusive arteriosclerosis of the lower limbs," *Pol. Tyg. Lek.* 1991;46(37-39):700-703

[5] A Romero Valdes et al., "Ozone therapy in the advanced stages of arteriosclerosis obliterans," *Angiologia* 1993; 45(4):146-148.

Chapter 15
Nature's Provision

[1] A Kalen et al. "Age-related changes in the lipid compositions of rat and human tissues", *Lipids* 24, (1989):579-581

[2] A Kontushi et al., "Plasma ubiquinol-10 is decreased in patients with hyperlipidaemia", *Atherosclerosis* 129, (1997):119-126.

K Folkers et al. "Evidence for a deficiency of coenzyme Q10 in human heart disease", *Int. J. Vitamin. Nutr. Res.* 40, (1970):380-390.

[3] E Baggio et al. "Italian multicenter study on the safety and efficacy on coenzyme Q10 as adjunctive therapy in heart failure. The CoQ10 Drug Surveillance Investigators," *Clin. Invest.* 71 (Suppl 8),(1993):S145-S149.

GS Wander et al. "Randomized, double-blind placebo-controlled trial of coenzyme Q10 in patients with acute myocardial infarction", *Cardiovascular Drugs and Therapy* 12, (1998):347-353.

[4] RB Singh and MA Niaz, "Serum concentration of lipoprotein(a) decreases on treatment with hydrosoluble coenzyme Q10 in patients with coronary artery disease: discovery of a new role", *International Journal of Cardiology* 68, (1999):23-29.

[5] AZ Reznick et al. "Antiradical effects in L-propionyl carnitine protection of the heart against ischemia-reperfusion injury: the possible role of iron chelation", *Arch Biochem. Biophys.* 296, (1992):394-401.

RB Singh et al, "A randomized, double-blind, placebo-controlled trial of L-carnitine in suspected acute myocardial infarction", *Postgrad. Med. Journal* 72, (1996):45-60.

[6] RN Iyer et al., "L-carnitine moderately improves the exercise tolerance in chronic stable angina," *J. Assoc. Physicians India* 48(11), (2000):1050-1052.

[7]   V Diglesi, et al, "L-carnitine adjuvant therapy in essential hypertension", *Clin. The.r* 5, (1994):391-395.

[8]   A Kobayashi et al., "L-carnitine treatment for congestive heart failure: Experimental and clinical study," *Japanese Circ. J.* 56,(1992):86-94.

[9]   M Maebashi et al., "Lipid lowering effect of carnitine in patients with type-IV Hyperlipoproteinaemia," *The Lancet* 2,(1978):805-807.

[10]   G Brevetti et al., "Propionyl-L-carnitine in intermittent claudication: Double-blind, placebo-controlled, dose titration, multicenter study", *Journal of the American College of Cardiology* 26, no.6 (1995):1411-1416.

[11]   J Arenas et al, "Carnitine in muscle, serum and urine of non-professional athletes: Effects of physical exercise, training, and L-carnitine administration", *Muscle and Nerve* 14, (1991):598-604.

[12]   The Investigators, "Study on propionyl-L-carnitine in chronic heart failure", *Eur. Heart* J. 20,(1999):70-76.

[13]   Mancini et al., "Controlled study on the therapeutic efficacy of propionyl-L-carnitine in patients with congestive heart failure," *Arzneimittelforschung* 42,(1992):1101-1104.

[14]   S. Iliceto et al., "Effect of L-carnitine administration on left ventricular remodeling after acute anterior myocardial infarction: The L-carnitine ecocardiografia digitalizzata infarto miocardio (CEDIM) trial," *J. of the Am. Coll. of Cardiol.* 26, no. 2(1995):380-387.

[15]   B Wittels, JF Spann, "Defective lipid metabolism in the failing heart", *Journal of Clinical Investigation* 47, (1968):1787-1794.

[16]   AZ Reznick et al. "Antiradical effects in L-propionyl carnitine protection of the heart against ischemia-reperfusion injury: the possible role of iron chelation", *Arch Biochem. Biophys.* 296, (1992):394-401.

[17]   RB Singh et al. "A randomized, double-blind, placebo-controlled trial of L-carnitine in suspected acute myocardial infarction", *Postgrad. Med. Journal* 72, (1996):45-60.

[18] AZ Reznick et al. "Antiradical effects in L-propionyl carnitine protection of the heart against ischemia-reperfusion injury: the possible role of iron chelation", *Arch Biochem. Biophys.* 296, (1992):394-401.

RB Singh et al. "A randomized, double-blind, placebo-controlled trial of L-carnitine in suspected acute myocardial infarction", *Postgrad. Med. Journal* 72, (1996):45-60.

[19] T Kamikawa et al., "Effects of L-carnitine on exercise tolerance in patients with stable angina pectoris", *Japanese Heart Journal* 25, (1984):587-597.

I Anand et al., "Acute and chronic effects of propionyl-L-carnitine on the hemodynamics, exercise capacity, and hormones in patients with congestive heart failure", Cardiovascular Drugs and Therapy 12, (1998):291-299.

G Brevetti et al., "Propionyl-L-carnitine in intermittent claudication: Double-blind, placebo-controlled, dose titration, multicenter study", *Journal of the American College of Cardiology* 26, no.6 (1995):1411-1416.

[20] N Awata et al. «Acute haemodyonamic effect of taurine on hearts in vivo with normal and depressed myocardial function», *Cardiovascular Research* 21, (1987):241–247.

[21] J Azuma et al. "Therapeutic effect of taurine in congestive heart failure: a double-blind crossover trial", *Clin. Cardiol* 8, no.5 (1985):276-282.

J Azuma. "Long-term effect of taurine in congestive heart failure: Preliminary report," In: R Huxtable *Taurine in Health and Disease* (New York: Plenum Press, 1994), 425-433.

[22] MJ Meldrum et al. "The effect of taurine on blood pressure, and urinary sodium, potassium and calcium excretion," In: R Huxtable and DV Michalk (eds), *Taurine in Health and Disease* (New York: Plenum Press, 1994), 207-215.

[23] A Sawamura et al. "Protection by oral pretreatment with taurine against the negative inotropic effects of low calcium medium on isolated perfused chick heart", *Cardiovascular Research* 17, (1983):620.

N Awata et al. "Acute haemodyonamic effect of taurine on hearts in vivo with normal and depressed myocardial

127

function", *Cardiovascular Research* 21, (1987):241-247.

[24] T Nakamura et al. "The protective effect of taurine on the biomembrane against damage produced by oxygen radicals", *Biol. Pharm. Bull.* 16, (1993):970-972.

[25] MJ Sole and KN Jeejebhoy, "Conditional nutritional requirements: therapeutic relevance to heart failure," *Herz* 27(2),(2002):174-178.

F Jeejebhoy et al., "Nutritional supplementation with Myo Vive repletes essential cardiac myocyte nutrients and reduces left ventricular size in patients with left ventricular dysfunction," *Am. Heart J.* 143(6),2002:1092-1100.

[26] CJ Holubarsch et al, "Survival and prognosis: investigation of Crataegeus extract WS 1442 in congestive heart failure (SPICE)-rationale, study design and study control," *Eur J. Heart Fail.* 2(4), (2000):431-437.

S Pöpping et al. "Effect of a hawthorn extract on contraction and energy turnover of isolated rat cardiomyocytes," *Arzneimittel-Forschung/Drug Research* 45(II), no, 11(1995):1157-1160.

[27] R Shanthi et al. "Effect of tincture of Crataegus on the LDL-Receptor activity of hepatic plasma membrane of rats fed an atherogenic diet", *Atherosclerosis* 123, (1996):235-241.

[28] N Reitbrock et al. "Actions of standardized extracts of Crataegus berries on exercise tolerance and quality of life in patients with congestive heart failure," *Arzneimittelforschung* 51(10), (2001):793-798.

[29] M Sato et al. «Cardioprotective effects of grape seed proanthocyanidin against ischemic reperfusion injury», *Journal of Molecular and Cellular Cardiology* 31, (1999):1289–1297.

[30] Sato et al. "Grape seed proanthocyanidin reduces cardiomyocyte apoptosis by inhibiting ischemia reperfusion-induced activation of JNK-1 and C-Jun," *Free Radical Biol. Med.* 31(6), (2001):729-737.

[31] M Carini et al. "Complexation of Ginkgo biloba extract with phosphatidylcholine improves cardioprotective activtity

128

and increases the plasma capacity in the rat," *Planta Med.* 67(4),(2001):326-330.

[32] K Welt and L Schaffranietz, "Myocardium—protective effects of Ginkgo biloba extract (EGb 761) in old rats against acute isobaric hypoxia. An electron microscopic morphometric study. II Protection of microvascular endothelium", *Exp. Toxic. Pathol.* 48, (1996):81–86.

[33] PF Smith et al., "The neuroprotective effect of the Ginkgo biloba leaf: A review of the possible relationship to platelet-activating factor (PAF)," *J. Etnopharmacol 50,* (1996):131-1239.

[34] DD Haines et al. "Cardioprotective effects of the calcineurin inhibitor FK506 and the PAF receptor antagonist and free radical sacavenger, EGb 761 in isolated ischemic/reperfused rat hearts," *J. Cardiovasc. Pharmacol.* 35(1),(2000):37-44.

[35] K Welt et al. «Myocardium—protective effects of Ginkgo biloba extract (EGb 761) in old rats against acute isobaric hypoxia. An electron microscopic morphometric study. II Protection of microvascular endothelium», *Exp. Toxic. Pathol.* 48, (1996):81–86.

[36] M Steiner et al. «A double-blind crossover study in moderately hypercholesterolemic men that compared the effect of aged garlic extract and placebo administration on blood lipids» *American Journal of Clinical Nutrition* 64, (1996):866–870.

[37] M Steiner and W Li, "Aged garlic extract, a modulator of cardiovascular risk factors: A dose-finding study in the effects of AGE on platelet functions," *J. Nutr.,* 131, (2001):980S-984S.

Yeh Y-Y and L Liu, "Cholesterol-lowering effect of garlic extracts and organosulfur compounds: Human and animal studies," *J. Nutr.,* 131, (2001):989S-993S.

[38] H Rene Malinow et al., «Homocysteine, diet, andc ardiovascular diseases,» American Heart Association, www.americanheart.org/Scientific/statements/1999/019901.html

[39] Ibid.

[40] S Hernandez-Diaz S et al. "Dietary folate and the risk of nonfatal myocardial infarction," *Epidemiology* 13(6), (2002):700-706.

[41] PL Canner et al., "Fifteen year mortality in coronary drug project patients: Long term benefit with niacin", *Journal of the American College of Cardiology* 8, (1986):1245-1255. MH Luria, "Effect of low-dose niacin on high density lipoprotein cholesterol and total cholesterol/high-density lipoprotein cholesterol ratio", *Archives of Internal Medicine* 148, (1998):2493-2495.

[42] EB Rimm et al. "Folate and vitamin B6 from diet and supplements in relation to risk of coronary heart disease among women", *Journal of the American Medical Association* 279, no.5 (1998):359-364.

[43] O Nygard et al. "Plasma homocysteine levels and mortality in patients with coronary artery disease," *New Eng. J. Med.* 337,(1997):230-236.

[44] MJ Stampfer et al., "A prospective study of plasma homocyst(e)ine and risk of myocardial infarction in US physicians", *Journal of the American Medical Association* 268, no.7 (1992):877-881.

[45] See note 42.

[46] L Ling et al., "Vitamin C preserves endothelial function in patients with coronary heart disease after a high-fat meal," *Clin. Cardiol.* 25(5),(2002):219-224.

[47] F Gao et al., "Enhancement of glutathione cardioprotection by ascorbic acid in myocardial reperfusion injury," *J. Pharmacol. Exp. Ther.* 301(2), (2002):543-550.

[48] H Thomas and II Maugh, «High Vitamin C Levels in Blood are Found Beneficial,» *Los Angeles Times,* 3/5/2001, S3.

[49] Ibid.

[50] SP Azen et al. "Effect of supplementary antioxidant vitamin intake on carotid arterial wall intima-media thickness in a controlled clinical trial of cholesterol lowering", *Circulation* 94, (1996):2369-2372.

[51] EB Rimm et al. «Vitamin E consumption and the risk of

coronary heart disease onset in men», *New England Journal of Medicine* 328, (1993):1450–1456.

[52] KK Witte et al. "Chronic heart failure and micronutrients," *J. Am. Coll. Cardiol.* 37(7),(2001):1765-1774.

[53] RP Heaney and MJ Barger-Lux , "Low calcium intake: the culprit in many chronic diseases," *J. Dairy Sci.* 77,(1994):1155-1160.

LJ Appel et al. "A clinical trial of the effects of dietary patterns on blood pressure," *New England Journal of Medicine* 336, (1997):1117-1124.

[54] Dwyer JH et al., "Dietary calcium, calcium supplementatiuon, and blood pressure in African American adolescents," *Am. J. Clin. Nutr.* 68,(1998):648-655.

[55] KN Jeejeebhoy, "The role of chromium in nutrition and therapeutics as a potential toxin," *Nutrition Rev.* 57(11), (1999):329-335.

[56] MF McCarty, Subtoxic intracellular trivalent chromium is not mutagenic: implications for safety of chromium supplementation," *Med. Hypotheses* 49(3),(1997):263-269.

[57] RI Press et al. "The effect of chromium picolinate on serum cholesterol and apolipoprotein fractions in human subjects", *The Western Journal of Medicine* 152, (1990):41-45.

JB Gordon , "An easy and inexpensive way to lower cholesterol?", *The Western Journal of Medicine* 154, (1991):352.

[58] M Simonoff et al. "Low plasma chromium in patients with coronary artery and heart disease", *Biol. Trace Elem Res.* 6, (1984):431-439.

[59] M Shechter et al. "Beneficial effects of magnesium sulfate in acute myocardial infarction", *American Journal of Cardiology* 66, (1990):271-274.

[60] Ibid.

[61] MS Neff, "Magnesium sulfate in digitalis toxicity", American Journal of Cardiology 29, (1972):377-382.

[62] L Ceremuzynski et al. "Hypomagnesemia in heart failure with ventricular arrhythmia: Beneficial effects of magnesium supplementation," *J. Intern. Med.* 247(1),(2000):78-86.

131

[63] PK Whelton et al. "Effects of oral potassium on blood pressure: Meta-analysis of randomized controlled clinical trials", *Journal of the American Medical Assocaitaion* 277, no.20 (1997):1624-1632.

[64] M Slama et al., "Prevention of Hypertension," Curr. Opin. Cardiol. 17(5), (2002):531-536.

[65] Barry Sears, Ph.D., *The Zone* (New York: HarperCollins) p. 114.

[66] Barry L. Zaret, *Yale University School of Medicine Heart Book* (New York: William Morrow and Company), pp. 281 and 141.

[67] Ibid. p. 145.

[68] Ibid, p. 243.

[69] Burton Goldberg. *Alternative Medicine. The definitive Guide.* (Tiburon,California: Future Medicine Publishing, Inc., 1999), 718.

Chapter 16
Heart On Your Sleeve

[1] P Artemis et al. *The Omega Plan*, (New York: HarperCollins), 1998, p. 96.

[2] Amy Norton, «Unhappy marriages may harm women's hearts,» 3/13/01. Reuters Ltd., Center for Cardiovascular Education, Inc. www.heartinfo.org

[3] «The second act of Dean Ornish,» by Bill Thomson, *Natural Health*, Nov.–Dec. 1998 www.findarticles.com/cf_0/m0NAH/n6_v27/21253049/p1/article.jhtml?term=

[4] 1/11/01, Page 1D, «Exercising may fight depression in the long run,» By Marilyn Elias, (c) Copyright 2000 *USA TODAY*, a division of Gannett Co. Inc.

[5] Tandas de Penales aumentan probabilidad de sufrir infartos, CNN, December 19, 2002, http://www.cnnenespañol.com?2002/salud/12/19/penales/index.html

APPENDIX I

About the Author

Francisco Contreras, MD is a conventionally trained medical doctor who has gained worldwide attention not so much for his refined skill as a cancer surgeon but more for his ostentatious ability to integrate natural therapies with orthodox medicine in pursuit of total well-being for his patients.

Dr. Contreras received international training beginning first with pre-med at Pasadena College, Pasadena, California. He went on to complete medical school and the Universidad Autonoma de Mexico in 1978. After a year of social medical service, he traveled with his new bride, Rosa Alicia Contreras to Vienna, Austria to specialize in surgical oncology at one of the world's finest medical schools the Chirurgeshe Univeritatslkink which is recognized for producing such renowned doctors as Dr. Sigmund Freud. Soon after completing his specialty, he returned to Mexico and began to work with his father at the Oasis of Hope Hospital in 1983.

With his recent release from one of the top medical schools in Europe, he was enthusiastic and ready to bring all of the latest information and techniques to his father and patients. He was eager to share his knowledge but quickly he realized that it was his father who was the deep pool of medical wisdom. As a child,

133

he had been around his father's medical practice constantly and he was aware of his father's professional excellence; but, as a physician, now a colleague of his father, he was amazed at the results his father was achieving with patients who had received no help from conventional medicine. Dr. Contreras became a student once again. It has now been twenty years since he began. In 1998, his father passed his torch to Dr. Contreras who now leads the team at Oasis of Hope in his father's total care approach to patient care.

Patients continue to come to the Oasis of Hope from around the world but Dr. Contreras is taking the experience of 40 years of medical practice with 100,000 patients to the world. He shares through television, radio and conferences including the World Conference On Breast Cancer. He has met with top officials including the Chairman of the Japanese FDA and the Georgia State House of Representatives.

Dr. Contreras believes that most people are falling to disease due to lack of knowledge. He believes that education has greater impact in improving the health of humanity than breakthroughs in the area of research. It is this conviction that compels him to travel extensively to share knowledge with those who will partake of it. As a part of his mission, he has authored nine books and has three books that are currently in process dealing with the themes cancer, joint health, menopause, anti-aging, the secret healing power contained within tomatoes, heart health and the modern day adversaries of health.

Dr. Contreras also founded the Francisco Contreras Clinical Research Organization (FCCRO) which is run under the direction of Dr. Jorge Baroso, MD, Ph.D. FCCRO has conducted a number of clinical trials, formulated unique natural food supplements and has designed protocols for clinical trials on new drugs. Currently it is in process of registering a blood substitute in Mexico. If successful, there will finally be an alternative to blood transfusions which are often tainted with disease such as hepatitis and

AIDS. The new blood substitute is sterile and will function with all blood types which is vital during times of blood shortage. FCCRO also compiles all of the research that Dr. Contreras needs for his books.

Dr. Contreras has registered Hope Humanitarian Projects with the mission of improving the quality of life of indigent people in Mexico through education, sewage and waste management and medical care. This non-profit group gives its support to a ministry that reaches out to inmates in twenty-two prisons throughout Mexico. It is also planning to work with another group that provides needed heart surgery on children who have no means of paying for the procedures.

With all of these projects and activities, it would seem that Dr. Contreras has very little time to spend with his family but he enjoys lunch with his beautiful wife and five children everyday at home and on the weekends, they are very active in sports including tennis, swimming, snow skiing, motorcycle racing and spinning. They attend church in San Diego, California at The Rock where the evangelist Miles McPherson preaches. His wife and children are involved in two ministries called Fundacion Emanuel which reaches out to women and Generacion Retos which reaches out to youth.

Dr. Contreras believes that every person has the right to information that will empower people to make correct health decisions. He also has great compassion and his patients often comment how warm and caring he is. He operates under the belief that his life does not belong to himself; rather, God has put him here to serve others. He is very outspoken that healing a patient's body is only a temporary solution but healing a person's soul is everlasting.

APPENDIX II

About the Oasis of Hope Hospital

Recently, *Newsweek* magazine featured an article about the new trend of American's choosing to seek alternative therapies to complement what their doctors are prescribing to them. A study from Harvard Medical School concluded that more than 50 percent of Americans are taking some type of complementary or alternative therapy. What is striking is that within the last ten years, the National Institutes of Health has increased the budget for researching alternative medicine from two million dollars annually to one hundred million dollars. The time has finally come in America where the establishment is no longer calling alternative methods quackery but now looking for ways to integrate them into mainstream medical practices.

Francisco Contreras' father, Dr. Ernesto Contreras, Sr., was at least 40 years ahead of his time. He opened the Oasis of Hope Hospital in 1963 with the purpose of ministering to the needs of the whole person – body, mind and spirit. He never abandoned conventional medicine. In fact, he was a pioneer in conventional medicine. After completing a fellowship in pediatric pathology at Boston Children's Hospital at Harvard, he became the very first pathologist in the northwest of Mexico and he was needed to serve hospitals in San Diego, California as well in the late 1950's.

Dr. Ernesto Contreras only had one objection to the traditional medicine he was schooled in. Its primary objective was to eradicate disease. Often times this would lead to very aggressive therapies that would harm the patient more than the disease. As a pathologist examining cells and tissue under the microscope, he became astounded at the number of unnecessary surgeries being performed and the number of misdiagnoses that were taking place. He came to the conclusion that these errors were due to the separation doctor's had with their patients. Doctors were instructed in medical school to keep from establishing personal relationships with patients to avoid risking their objectivity. But Dr. Contreras felt that the only way to determine the true problems and needs of the patient was to get to know everything about the patient. He changed his medical objective from eradicating disease to providing physical, emotional and spiritual resources according to the needs of the patient to bring the patient back into balance allowing the body to heal itself. He often found that what a patient needed was not a drug but maybe minerals or vitamins. He also noted that a depressed person would respond better to the treatment if he had sessions of laughter therapy and counseling. The practice of music, laughter and prayer therapy combined with a nutrition program and natural therapies gained the Oasis of Hope Hospital, a conventional hospital, a reputation as an alternative hospital. That was never the goal and it is not quite accurate. The Oasis of Hope provides integrative medicine which is to say a combination of conventional and alternative medicine. Dr. Contreras states that it is not important what treatment is used. The important thing is why and when a specific treatment is used. The medical decisions made by the doctors at the Oasis of Hope are made complying with the principles established by founder, Dr. Ernesto Contreras. Sr.

Principles

I. Do No Harm

II. Love Your Patient As Yourself

137

These principles may seem simple but they have a profound impact. Why? Oasis physicians ask themselves two questions before they prescribe any medication or therapy.

1. Will this medication I wish to prescribe harm the patient or cause side effects that are unreasonable to have and tolerate for the benefit that it will give in return?

2. If I had the same condition, would I take the medication I wish to prescribe to this patient? Does the medical literature, my experience and the counsel of my peers indicate that this medication has a high probability of helping the patient?

These questions are especially important for oncologists to ask themselves. Chemotherapy is the most common cancer treatment prescribed to cancer patients yet the medical literature indicates that it is effective in very few types of cancer. If you talk to patients taking chemotherapy, they will tell you that the side effects are unbearable. And to top it all off, very few oncologists are willing to take chemotherapy themselves.

Cancer Treatment at Oasis of Hope

Dr. Contreras operates a beautiful modern medical/surgical hospital fully equipped with everything you would expect at a world-class facility including digital diagnostic equipment, intensive care unit, emergency services and highly trained medical staff. The physicians are versed in conventional cancer therapy and able to utilize chemotherapy, radiation and surgery in limited cases when it is in the best interest of the patient.

But Dr. Contreras is most known for using non-conventional cancer therapies. The most famous of which are laetrile, shark cartilage, Emulsified Vitamin A and Extra-corporeal Systemic Oxygenation.

Laetrile (Vitamin B-17/Amygdalin)

Laetrile (also called Vitamin B-17 and Amygdalin) is a powerful and natural anti-tumor agent. Laetrile is a natural chemothera-

138

peutic agent found in over 1,200 plants, particularly in the seeds of common fruits such as apricots, peaches, plums and apples. It is a diglucoside with a cyanide radical that is highly "bio-accessible." This means that it penetrates through the cellular membrane, reaching high intra-cellular concentrations easily. Normal cells in the body contain an enzyme called rhodenase which "neutralizes" the laetrile. This enzyme prevents the laetrile from releasing cyanide. Laetrile serves as glucose to healthy cells that provides energy when metabolized.

Malignant cells do not contain the rhodenase enzyme. In the absence of rhodenase, laetrile is activated and the cyanide radical is released within malignant cells. The end result is tumor destruction. The wonderful thing about laetrile is that it only affects cancerous cells and normal cells are left unharmed.

As laetrile attacks unhealthy cells, it transforms into a salicilate which is much like aspirin. It contributes greatly to pain control. Laetrile is extremely effective in the prevention of a cancer relapse. Because laetrile is natural and non-toxic, it can be taken at a lower dosage for life as a preventative therapy.

Recent studies indicate that cyanide may be the most powerful anti-cancer agents nature has to offer. A group of scientists in the Department of Biochemistry at London's Imperial College have developed a way to treat cancer called Antibody-Directed Enzyme Pro-Drug Therapy (ADEPT). This approach utilizes cancer seeking anti-bodies as a shuttle that can deliver anti-cancer agents right to the malignant cell. The scientists are using cyanide as the anti-cancer agent which is exactly the same as is found in laetrile. One of the scientists working on this project at London's Imperial College told Dr. Contreras, "We have demonstrated that this system [ADEPT] is able to specifically kill tumor cells by cyanide intoxication." Now in the new millennium, science is catching up with what Dr. Ernesto Contreras, Sr. pioneered four decades ago.

Shark Cartilage
Shark cartilage inhibits the growth of blood vessels which feed growing tumors, thereby restricting the vitality of the tumor. In other words, it is an antiangiogenesis agent. This is a non-toxic product which increases the production of antibodies within the immune system. It is recommended for cancer and other inflammatory diseases.

In a clinical trial conducted by Dr. Contreras and Dr. Lane, it was noted that tumors frequently experience significant reduction in size within one to three months of the initial treatment. It was also noted to enhance the efficacy of laetrile.

Emulsified Vitamin A
Emulsified Vitamin A is accepted as an agent of great use in important cancer centers, most of all, on epidermoid carcinomas, chronical leukemia and transitional cells.

Extra-Corporeal Systemic Oxygenation
Dr. Otto Warburg demonstrated that malignant cells proliferate in an anaerobic environment whereas normal cells require oxygen to survive. The solution to cancer seems simple – introduce oxygen directly to the malignant cells. If only it were that easy. Tumors have a mechanism that reduces the presence of oxygen within them which causes the cells lining the inside of blood vessels (endothelial cells) to release "Vascular Endothelial Growth Factor" (VEGF). VEGF stimulates the reproduction of blood vessels. The increase in blood vessels allows tumors to grow. As the number of blood vessels around tumors increase, they become restricted or collapse which also makes it very difficult for oxygen or even cancer drugs to reach the tumor. This is the ideal condition for unrestricted multiplication of malignant cells.

Many different ways have been devised to deliver oxygen to tumors. The inhalation consumption, infusion or insufflations of oxygen, ozone and hydrogen peroxide in liquid and gas forms have met with limited success. Mechanical delivery systems such as tubes, needles and respirators have not produced sufficient results. What has been required is a biochemical delivery system. In order for oxygen to penetrate tumors, it must be converted into ozone (O_3), introduced into the bloodstream where it converts to hydrogen peroxide (H_2O_2), that reaches the inner layers of the blood vessels which causes them to dilate allowing oxygen to pass into ischemic areas such as tumors. Why not introduce O_2 instead of O_3? O_2 does not create the biochemical reaction needed. Why not infuse H_2O_2? The required doses of H_2O_2 to make the biochemical mechanism function are toxic.

Mechanism of Action

O_3 therapy is completely non-toxic because the O_3 induces the beneficial biochemical mechanism without producing an undesirable residue or byproduct. O_3 decomposes in the blood water and reacts immediately with several substances generating a cascade of reactive oxygen species such as H_2O_2 that have longer lifetimes than ozone and if unquenched penetrate blood cells. Owing to the fact that blood is a sort of universe containing so many different cells and compounds, it has become possible to understand why ozonated blood displays different biological and therapeutic activities.

First, when H_2O_2 penetrates red cells and endothelial cells (the inner lining of blood vessels) it leads to 1) an increase in delivery and release of oxygen by hemoglobin toward the tissues (including tumors), 2) an increase in vasodilatation in ischemic areas and reduction of hypoxia (this means that oxygen penetrates tumors), and 3) an inhibition of the formation of new blood vessels due to the improvement of oxygenation of the neoplastic tissue due to ozone's action, thus restraining tumor growth.

Second, when H_2O_2 penetrates leukocytes, it induces the production of a special type of substance called cytokines such as interferon, interleukin and others, which can stimulate an array of

141

immune functions such as activation of macrophages and neutrophils which retard the cancer progression in immuno-depressed patients.

Third, an exciting new aspect is that ozone, being a strong oxidizer, stimulates efficiency of antioxidant systems in the long term. Usually after six to ten sessions of introducing O_3 into the bloodstream, cells begin to experience relief from oxidative stress. These findings may have an important practical implication because aging, chronic viral infections, cancer, and autoimmune and neurodegenerative diseases are accompanied by a pro-oxidant state with a progressive decay of intracellular detoxification so that the system of reduction-oxidation becomes unbalanced (towards oxidation).

O_3 treatment also eliminates viruses, bacteria and fungus which also relieves a burden from the immune system allowing for faster recovery from illness.

Anti-tumor properties of O_3 thus depend on O_3 concentration and length of exposure. All these effects have an O_3 dose threshold and there is also a toxicity threshold. Between the two, there is a window in which ozone could have therapeutic effects. The sudden rise of H_2O_2 in the cytoplasm must reach a certain threshold in order to activate biochemical pathways, and this implies that if the dose O_3 is too low, no activation will ensue and only a placebo effect could take place. On the other hand, if the H_2O_2 level is too high owing to an inappropriately excessive O_3 dose, the specter of oxidation and the damage to vital intracellular components occur.

The Oasis physicians utilize an extra corporeal loop much like that used for kidney dialysis. An O_3 generator is attached to the loop and the flow rate of O_3, blood saturation level and duration are monitored and controlled. The patient's entire blood volume is exposed to O_3 for the duration that is required and the oxygen levels in the bloodstream may be increased up to 650 percent if necessary. The experience at the Oasis of Hope of introducing O_3 into the bloodstream has produced favorable objective results in many patients and complete eradication of cancer in a number of patients.

Results

The Oasis of Hope conducts retrospective studies periodically to document the five-year survival rates of its cancer patients. It is important to note that 95 percent of these patients had stage IV cancers (this means that the cancer had spread from the primary site to another organ) after conventional therapy had failed to help them. These patients were treated with Contreras metabolic therapy and the results were encouraging. The overall five-year survival rate for all types of cancer was 30 percent. The study also noted that 86 percent of the patients outlived their prognosis and reported an improvement in their quality of life.

Malignancies in the lung, breast, colon and prostate are the most prevalent. For this reason, the study focused on the efficacy of metabolic therapy in these advanced stage IV cancers. In the table below, the Oasis patient's results are compared against those from clinical trials with conventional therapies.

TYPE OF CANCER DISTANT[1]	NUMBER OF PATIENTS	5 YR. SURVIVAL RATE (%)	
		OASIS	CONVENTIONAL[2]
Lung Cancer	200	30%	2%
Breast Cancer	130	39%	21%
Colon Cancer	150	30%	8%
Prostate Cancer	600	86%	33%

1. Distant: A malignant cancer that has spread to parts of the body remote from the primary tumor either by direct extension or by discontinuous metastasis to distant organs, tissues, or via the lymphatic system to distant lymph nodes.
2. Source: American Cancer Society Cancer Facts & Figures 2001

143

The Oasis statistics when compared to the Conventional statistics are dramatically better. What makes these results astounding is the difference between the Oasis group and the Conventional group. The Oasis patients had already undergone surgery, radiation or chemotherapy. They had endured the hair loss, nausea, burns and devastation of their energy levels and immune systems. Those in the Conventional group had no previous treatment to damage their general condition. They had a fresh start.

If you would like more information about cancer treatment at the Oasis of Hope Hospital, please call toll free 1-888-500-HOPE and visit the Internet site: **www.oasisofhope.com.**

Oasis of Hope Hospital
PO BOX 439045
San Ysidro, CA 92143
Tel: (888) 500-HOPE
Tel: (619) 690-8450
Fax: (619) 690-8410
Internet: www.oasisofhope.com
Email: health@oasisofhope.com

APPENDIX III
Cholesterol Ratios

Your cholesterol ratios should be as follows:

Total Cholesterol/HDL=<4

LDL/HDL=<3

To calculate your ratios, have a blood test and ask for them to measure your total cholesterol, your HDL and your LDL levels. Then plug those numbers into the formula:

Your total cholesterol____/your HDL____=

Your LDL____/your HDL____ =

If the first number is 4 or more and/or the second number is 3 or above, you are considered to be at high risk of cardiovascular disease and should consult a physician as soon as possible.

For more information, please visit www.nutritionfacts.us

APPENDIX IV
Body Mass Index (BMI)

How to calculate your body mass index.
All you need to do is fill in the blanks and use your calculator.
1. Weigh yourself in pounds.
2. Measure yourself in inches.
3. Multiply your weight by 705.
4. Divide that result by your height in inches.
5. Divide the new result by your height again and that number will be your BMI.

Formula:
Your weight_____ X 705 = Z
Z/Your height in inches _____= Y
Y/Your height in inches = Your BMI =____

If your BMI is between 18.5 and 25, you are considered to be healthy.

If your BMI is between 25 and 30, you are considered to be overweight with moderate risk for heart problems. If your BMI is over 30 you are considered to be at high risk. Whatever your BMI is, you should consult your doctor and have your heart health checked out.

146

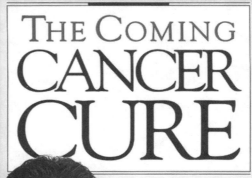

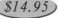
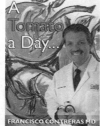
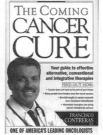
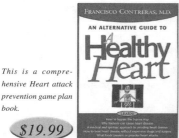
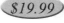
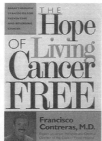
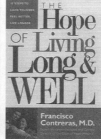
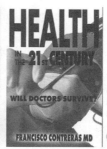

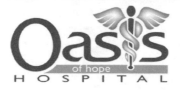
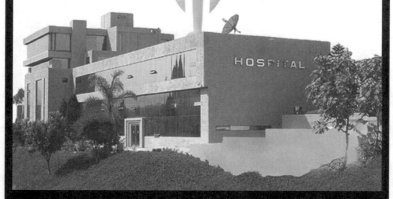

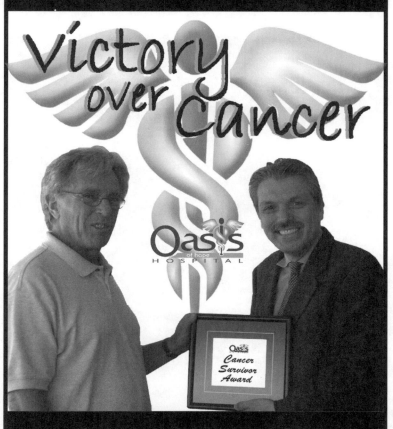